Ask the Chiropractor II

Ask the Chiropractor II

Steven J. Pollack, D.C.

iUniverse, Inc.
New York Lincoln Shanghai

Ask the Chiropractor II

iUniverse books may be ordered through booksellers or by contacting:

iUniverse
2021 Pine Lake Road, Suite 100
Lincoln, NE 68512
www.iuniverse.com
1-800-Authors (1-800-288-4677)

ISBN-13: 978-0-595-37366-6 (pbk)
ISBN-13: 978-0-595-81763-4 (ebk)
ISBN-10: 0-595-37366-6 (pbk)
ISBN-10: 0-595-81763-7 (ebk)

Printed in the United States of America

Dedicated to those who remind me that the giving and receiving of love supercedes all else in life.

Contents

How to benefit from these columns xiii

Adjustments are based on need, not time 1

Allergy sufferers need heightened immune system 2

American's perception of health is faulty 4

Anomalies are evident in many patients 6

Antibiotic overuse 8

Antibiotics and ear infections 10

Athletic ointments give temporary relief 11

Avoid self adjustments 13

Babies need brain/body coordination 14

Baby boomers fear decreased physical activity as they age 16

Back pain relief linked to combination of Chiropractic and
    exercise 18

Beach chairs can irritate back conditions 19

Be aware of early warning signs of poor health 21

Bitter is better when it comes to fruits and vegetables 23

Breast-feeding helps infant eczema 25

Breast-feeding is best for newborns 27

Cause of fatigue may be self evident 28

Chiropractic can help you prevent the flu this winter. 30

Chiropractic, diet, and exercise assist blood pressure conditions. 32

Chiropractic helps children 34

Chiropractic is a family affair. 36

Chiropractic is a mainstream healing profession. 38

Chiropractic is recognized around the world 40

Chiropractors become unified 42

Chiropractors hold the key to anti-aging 44

Chiropractors take aim at educating the public 45

Combined stretching and strengthening best management for
    low back 47

Conquer your accident fears 49

Discuss destructive health habit changes with your doctor. 51

Don't underestimate your brain. 53

Drug ads directed to consumer, not physicians 55

Early detection of postural changes in children allows proper
    growth 57

Early to bed kids are healthier 60

Education is essential for healthy patient 62

Environment can influence health 64

Everyone gets vertebral subluxations 66

Excess video-game playing can injure wrists. 68

Excessive TV watching can be hazardous to a child's health. 70

Exercise best therapy for chronic fatigue 72

Explain your pain 74

Extra vertebra is a common anomaly. 76

Fibromyalgia linked to fatigue syndrome. 78

Follow Mother Theresa's lead 80

Forgiveness is healing 82

Give yourself the gift of Chiropractic 83

Grieving is normal and healthy 85

Head and facial injuries require immediate attention. 87

High heels are a potential hazard. 89

High heels can cause knee problems 90

Holistic health care is choice care of 21st century 91

How we stand has a direct effect on our spines 93

How you carry pocketbook can create neck and/or back pain 94

Hypochondriacs can be helped with group therapy. 96

Infant care—safe and smart. 98

Innate intelligence and Chiropractic 100

Insurance coding complicated procedure. 102

Jet lag helped by Chiropractic care 104

Laughter heals. 105

Love heals 106

Lumbar-support belts stabilize the low back 108

Many "myths" about low-back pain 110

Massage and Chiropractic enter mainstream 112

Medical and Chiropractic philosophies differ drastically 114

Medicare covers Chiropractic 116

Mid-back pain is a serious condition 117

Mood swings helped by Chiropractic care 119

Movement for infants is vital 121

Musicians must be careful of posture 123

Nation is getting sicker 125

Natural sunlight is healthier than artificial 127

Neck and head injuries are severe. 129

Nerve conduction testing is beneficial diagnostic tool 131

Nerve injuries cause immune system suppression. 132

Nutrition and Chiropractic are good alternatives to hormone
    replacement. 134

Osteoporosis helped by Chiropractic 136

Overuse of painkillers can cause pain 138

Pain can be transferred to opposite ends of the spine 140

Pain-killer medications have high risk for back-pain control 142

Pain thresholds vary due to natural chemicals 144

Pets help heal their owners. 146

Poor eating habits damage health. 148

Potential law suits mean more paperwork 150

Preparation prevents sports injuries 152

Prepare prior to morning stretching. 154

Prevention is best policy to avoid injuries around the house. 156

Proper positioning prevents back pain while driving 158

Protect yourself from antibiotics 160

Psoas muscles keep our lower spine straight 162

Quality-of-life progress best assessed by patient 164

Reason for X-rays 166

Rib pains take time to heal 168

Roller-coaster rides 170

Sciatica—Chiropractic best treatment 171

Scooter injuries on the rise 173

Seat-belt whiplash 174

Seek care immediately with back pain 176

Self-help tips to help harness chronic headaches 178

Sick and tired of being sick and tired? 180

Side effects from adjustments are rare 181

Simple healthy dieting guidelines 183

Sleep position for back health 185

Smoking increases low-back pain 187

Spenoid bone stabilizes the skull 188

Spinal stretching reduces back pain 189

Spine develops first and controls all functions 191

State Workers' Compensation laws need changes 193

Straight look at curve balls 195

Summer sports require warm ups 197

Tai Chi is the perfect exercise for elderly 199

Teeth grinding at night is a sign of imbalance 201

Tennis elbow solution 203

Tingling/numb extremities have multiple causes 204

Tips to stay young in your 40s 206

Tubes for ear infections may be avoided 207

U.S.A. has a mental-health crisis 209

Visualization therapy 211

Vitamin supplement content can be deceiving 213

Weekend warrior 214

Whiplash can occur from injuries other than auto accidents 216

You can prevent your own back pain 218

Youth back pain common, but not normal 220

How to benefit from these columns

I. Public relations

1. Start your own column in local papers.

    a. Make your face familiar to the public.

    b. Repetition sells in marketing

2. Reference columns for patient education.

    a. Save time in explanation. Time for more patients.

    b. Educate your staff.

3. Open doors by validating yourself as an established professional in the community.

    a. Use columns in mailings.

    b. Use columns in portfolio to obtain lectures and events in your community.

4. Education of your community, friends, family, and employees.

5. Web-site promotions and E-mail lists.

II. Personal growth

A. Create your own question and answer columns besides existing questions and answers in this book.

B. Stay in touch with everything happening in the Chiropractic profession.

C. Express yourself. Be heard by thousands in your community.

D. Maintain your philosophical beliefs.

E. E. Increase listening skills to grasp new ideas and questions on health from patients, employees, friends, and family.

III. Our profession

A. Your time is a gift back to the profession.

B. Expand the circle of knowledge. Inspire new well-grounded students of Chiropractic.

Adjustments are based on need, not time

Question: Why does my Chiropractor only take a few minutes on my adjustment on some days and 10 minutes or more on others?

Answer: Chiropractic adjustments were originally designed to correct any neurological dysfunction that existed in the patient's spine on that day's treatment. The primary focus of all Chiropractors is to remove subluxations from the spine. Subluxations are misalignments of the vertebra that create interference to the function of that nerve route that exits between the two vertebra. The result of a subluxation will be a dysfunction to wherever that nerve enervates its cells, tissues, or organs. Although there may not be a symptom initially or even for extended times, it will always cause either too much or too little nerve supply to its destination. The job of your Chiropractor is to detect these subluxations and correct them. On any given day or in any stressful situation your nervous system an be overtaxed, resulting in subluxations. It is not only physical trauma that creates subluxations. It can be chemical, mental, job, family, or any combination of stressors that can contribute to neurological dysfunction.

Depending on your stress-load that day, or the amount of subluxations you have, will determine the amount of time your Chiropractor will have to spend with you. Your entire spine, as well as all structures in your body, work together and must be evaluated every visit. The key to a great adjustment is the quality of time your Chiropractor spends with you as well as how specific he or she can be in correcting your subluxations.

Quote of the week: *"It isn't where you came from; it's where you're going that counts."*—Ella Fitzgerald

Allergy sufferers need heightened immune system

Question: It is almost allergy season and I am already dreading going outside. What can I do to stop my allergy reactions this year?

Answer: Let's define what an allergy is first. Allergic reactions occur when the body perceives allergens (whatever the body is reacting to) as poison. When the body malfunctions and registers pollen, dust etc. as toxic, the immune system secretes a defense chemical called histamine. When histamine is released, the lining of the nose begins to swell. Symptoms may include watery, itchy eyes, runny nose, sneezing, swelling of the sinuses causing congestion, and heavy pressure headaches.

The real question is why some people react to the allergens while others exposed to the exact same allergens have no ill effects. The answer is that the immune system is directly connected to the nervous system. When the body is exposed to allergens it sends immediate messages to the brain to combat these invaders. If the immune system is suppressed or over taxed by other destructive activity, it will not be able to balance the effect of the invaders.

A major cause of disrupted pathways that carry communications to and from the brain to the immune system is a vertebral subluxation. A vertebral subluxation is where the spinal vertebrae are misaligned or fixated out of their normal position. The delicate nerves, which run the channels in the spinal column, can become irritated or compressed and unable to communicate information correctly. This theory explains why the immune system reads pollen as poison. The information isn't being transmitted correctly.

Fixing the misaligned vertebrae may fix the allergic reactions that are causing you so much pain and trouble. Chiropractors specialize in correcting vertebral subluxations. I am sure you could predict what my suggestion to you is for preventing a bad allergy season this year.

Quote of the week: *"A moment's insight is sometimes worth a life's experience."*—Oliver Wendell Holmes

American's perception of health is faulty

Question: I am confused as to what is considered healthy. My neighbor does 20 minutes of exercise 3-days a week but eats like a horse and is 50 pounds overweight and she claims she is healthy. How can this be?

Answer: American's have a misconception about what is healthy. Due to massive media propaganda, appearance and superficial beauty has been misunderstood to mean health. Many Americans wait until they are actively sick before they will consider themselves unhealthy. Many see the definition of healthy as, "I feel fine." This is a dangerous notion that needs to be replaced by the understanding that a person is healthy only when he or she is living a healthy lifestyle that is regularly monitoring key risk factors such as blood pressure and spinal function. Exercise is important but overtaxing a potentially critical organ or joint without acknowledging it's warning signs can be lethal.

A recent survey of 1,004 adults showed that 67 percent reported being physically active and only 30 percent perceived themselves as being overweight. The reality of our population based on statistics from the Department of Health and Human Services show 60 percent of Americans do not get enough physical activity to yield health benefits and that more than 25 percent are not active at all. In addition the statistics indicate that 64 percent of Americans are overweight. This is deplorable that two-thirds of our population is overweight and still feel like they are healthy. The first step in correcting a problem is admitting that you have one.

If you are not the one overweight and unhealthy this means the two people next to you probably are. I want education programs that teach wellness initiatives and incentives that encourage healthy life styles. Our next generations are already in severe health predicaments due to lack of exercise and horrific diets. Look at yourself in the mirror and be honest about your health. Change your life to a healthy lifestyle for yourself and the model you represent to our youth.

Quote of the week: *"America is a willingness of the heart."*—F. Scott Fitzgerald

Anomalies are evident in many patients

Question: My Chiropractor said I have spinal anomalies. What are anomalies and how do they affect me?

Answer: Anomalies are changes in the spine that are different than normal. Most patients demonstrate some type of anomaly on radiographs (X-rays). A study done in New Zealand and published in the *Journal of Manipulative and Physiological Therapies,* Nov./Dec. issue, listed the five most frequently occurring spinal anomalies found on spinal radiographs. They were in descending order: degenerative joint disease, posterior ponticle (a bone growth off the first cervical vertebra), soft-tissue abnormalities, transitional segments, and spondylolisthesis.

Each spinal change has a different effect on each individual. Most bony growth changes are either congenital or arthritic in orientation. A bony growth development can potentially irritate adjacent soft tissue or nerves, creating inflammation and pain. Soft tissue anomalies can irritate muscle and ligament functions. A spondylolisthesis which is a forward displacement of one vertebra on another, secondary to a fracture of the pars interarticularis (bilateral joints of the spine), can effect the lumbar spine by making it unstable. The range of symptoms secondary to a spondylolisthesis range from no problems to severe pain and instability.

Your physician should analyze all anomalies. Additional X-rays, magnetic resonance imaging's (MRI's) or diagnostic testing may be advised to further isolate and diagnose the possible dangers or causes that particular anomaly may have on that individuals function.

Chiropractors are well trained in administering and analyzing spinal radiographs. It is part of your Chiropractor's job to discuss the results of your films with you and the implications of their findings.

Quote of the week: *"Vision is the art of seeing things invisible."*—Jonathan Swift

Antibiotic overuse

Question: I have had an upper-respiratory infection for the entire winter. In previous years I took antibiotics, but this year nothing is helping me, in fact I feel worse. What can I do?

Answer: We are in a crisis as a nation regarding the substantial value that antibiotics have in preventing and killing bacterial origin disease. Penicillin given as 40,000 units a day for four days would destroy pneumococcal pneumonia in 1941. Today you could take 24-million units of penicillin a day and still die of pneumococcal meningitis.

D. Harold C. Neu, of Columbia University in New York states that, "Bacteria that cause infection of the respiratory tract, skin, bladder, bowel, and blood are now resistant to virtually all of the older antibiotics. The extensive use of antibiotic in the community and hospitals has fueled the crisis."

Bacteria develop resistance to drugs when exposed to them for extended periods. Bacteria can also pass the genes for resistance from one type to another. A sort of information super-highway exists among bacteria that allows resistance to spread rapidly among bacteria that have not even been exposed to a particular antibiotic. These and other factors have caused medicine to take a halting look at the current way in which antibiotics are used.

It is time we treat the person, not necessarily the bacteria. It is more likely that your immune system is compromised in some manner, making you more susceptible to infection. Diet, nutrition, lifestyle, environment, social and psychological factors all influence the immune system in significant ways. When unfavorable changes occur in these areas, immune function may suffer and bacteria may more easily proliferate.

Chiropractors correct subluxations which research indicates severely deters immune function. A balanced nervous system means a better balanced immune system.

More or better antibiotics are not the solutions. Re-evaluate all areas of your life to determine where there may be a chronic stress. If you are getting the same disease state every year, you are obviously conditioned either mentally, physically or chemically. You probably hold the key to the cause of your re-occurring illness and if you look close enough you can get better grasp of it.

Quote of the week: *"Our greatest fortune lies in our inner vault. Within is everything we could ever need."*—Anonymous

Antibiotics and ear infections

Question: My child gets a lot of ear infections. Are antibiotics needed for all his ear infections? I have heard all kinds of information that they may even make my child's condition worse. Is this true?

Answer: For decades, Chiropractors have expressed concern about the aggressive use of antibiotics in children with ear infection. Now, a study in the *British Medical Journal* validates that concern.

A total of 315 children diagnosed with acute Otitis Media (inner ear infection) were assigned to 1 of 2 cohorts: 1) a 72-hour waiting period with no antibiotic use or 2) immediate antibiotic intervention. Findings showed that "immediate anti-biotic prescription provided symptomatic benefit mainly after the first 24 hours, when symptoms were already resolving." Although children who were given antibiotics recovered an average of one day earlier than children who did not take the medication, no difference was seen in school absence or pain/distress scores. Another finding demonstrated 99-percent of children in the watchful waiting group developed diarrhea, compared with 19-percent of those taking anti-biotics.

The final outcome was that 77-percent of parents of children in the watchful waiting group expressed satisfaction with the care their youngsters received. In addition, these parents were less likely than parents of children who received antibiotics to predict that their youngsters would require antibiotics for subsequent ear infections.

Quote of the week: *"Do not let what you cannot do interfere with what you can do."*—John Wooden

Athletic ointments give temporary relief

Question: Do athletic lotions with icy/hot effects help heal injured muscles and joints?

Answer: Athletic lotions come in many different shapes and sizes with many different ingredients. In the old days Vicks Vapor Rub was all there was until Ben Gay came along. These products contained strong odors of menthol and gave a superficial skin sensation of heat. Modern era ointments contain many herbs, natural extracts and essential oils. Mineral Ice and Biofreeze are common ointments used in athletic-related injuries. They supply a sensation of both icy and hot simultaneously. Tiger Balm supplies a deep penetrating feeling of heat.

The temporary sensation of relief given by all these potions and lotions is just that, temporary relief. They do not replace appropriate therapies nor do they supply the equivalent effect as using ice packs or moist heat. These creams, ointments, rubs, etc. can last from 15 minutes to 4 hours depending on the type and amount utilized. Persistant pain, swelling and irritation should not be overlooked and you should consult your personal physician before using these analgesic products. There can be a detrimental effect if the ointments are used improperly. I have observed patience become dependent on these analgesics by using them throughout the day for weeks. The majority of conditions that do respond favorable are muscle and ligament sprains and strains. Remember my favorite acronym RICE when initially injuring a muscle, ligament or joint: RICE. R = Rest, I = Ice, C = Compression, E = Elevation. Do this for the first 48 hours following an injury and you will reduce pain and inflammation significantly. When ice, heat, and ointments don't reduce the extent of your injury, see your Chiropractor to get a proper exam, diagnosis and treatment.

Quote of the week: *"The man who has no imagination has no wings."*—Muhammad Ali

Avoid self adjustments

Question: My son is constantly cracking his own neck. Besides being annoying, is this damaging his spine?

Answer: Repetitive and excessive forceful cracking of any joint of the spine can lead to a stress injury overtime. Unnatural movement of the facet joints (the spinal articulations) can create inflammation in that area.

The need to constantly "crack" your own neck is usually due to the fact it feels uncomfortable. The irritation reappears because doing it to yourself doesn't correct the condition of spinal tension. Our office treats neck conditions, more commonly found in teenage patients that have the habit of repetitive cracking. Over stretching the joints irritates surrounding soft, tissue (ligament and muscles) and may make the joint hyper-mobile. The increased movement can prevent stability in the vertebral joint causing it to misalign and eventually subluxate (create neurological irritation). When the vertebral subluxation complex is created, Chiropractic adjustments are the most appropriate treatment.

Quote of the week: *"Those who bring sunshine to the lives of others cannot keep it from themselves."*—James Barrie

Babies need brain/body coordination

Question: My baby is not as coordinated in motor skills as the other babies in his play group. Could there be something wrong and what can I do?

Answer: Babies develop at very different speeds regarding motor skill development. Your baby is most likely fine, but there are definite means in which you can encourage and help develop these skills for your child. An article in *USA Today* discussed the guidelines issued by the National Association for Sport and Physical Activity concerning activity as a key factor in baby's motor skill development. In summary, they said that targeted daily activities are the building block for babies and toddlers for future tasks including walking, running, and playing.

We can't assume skills such as rolling, sitting, and walking will just come naturally as babies grow. There is a brain/body connection that needs to be stimulated. The study recommended the following guidelines:

Part of an infant's day should be spent in structured activity.

• Don't keep infant/toddlers in baby seats or other restrictive settings for a long time.

• Toddlers should accumulate at least 30-minutes of structured physical activity, and preschoolers at least an hour, each day.

• Toddlers and preschoolers should spend an hour or more a day in free play.

• Toddlers and preschoolers should not be sedentary for more than an hour at a time except when sleeping.

The guidelines imply that T.V. time for our future generation needs to be minimized and interactive organized and free-play expression time maximized. I am totally supportive of these guidelines. Your initial formation of active organized motor skills with your baby will reap big rewards, as your child gets older and more independent. Besides better coordination, your child will be more active and have a less chance of being over weight. Obesity in our children is in epidemic proportion. Starting the children with brain body functions will prevent future sedentary inactivity. Should your child continue to show signs of being slow at motor skills, appropriate childcare physicians can test him.

Quote of the week: *"The only difference between adults and children is the size of their sandbox."*—Anonymous

Baby boomers fear decreased physical activity as they age

Question: I have recently celebrated my 50th birthday and after reviewing my future concerns, realize that my biggest fear is not being able to physically perform in all areas of my life. What preventative or maintenance procedures can I perform now to prolong my physical fitness and health?

Answer: A market study done by Sage Products and published in *USA Today* statistically demonstrated that adults ages 37 to 55 say their biggest concern about growing old is slowing down physically. You are not alone. The health consciousness of this same age group, what I consider the heart and soul of the baby boomers, is focused directly on longevity with the highest potential health.

Unless you have been living in a cave, you will observe a mass media blitz focused on the baby boomers. Vitamins, minerals, hair-care products, weight loss, youth enhancements, and over-40 abdominal flattening (6 pack guaranteed) products are floating through your brain visually on TV, billboards, magazines and all day in your ears on the radio stations. Even if you perceive yourself as healthy, attractive, and fit, after this media blitz you start to question yourself. Don't be fooled by airbrushes and fast talking salesman. We are unfolding a new generation of health conscious parents.

The consensus of the baby-boomers concerns about aging resulted in these stats:

- slowing down physically—83 percent,

- overall health—81 percent,

- retirement/finances—69 percent,

- becoming a family burden—56 percent,

- caring for an ill spouse—54 percent, and

- having someone to care for them—54 percent.

Considering activity and health are the primary concerns of your future and the majority of others your age. Let me suggest the following basic principals. The number-one way to stay in shape is to stay active physically every day. Get a routine where you stretch or exercise every joint. Movement flushes dead stationary tissue out of joints, revitalizing the joint with fresh fluids full of minerals and vitamins. This prevents arthritis. Next, get enough sleep and eat sensible. Stay away from dense carbohydrates such as rice, pasta, bread, and corn. Increase your water intake to 4 to 6, 12 oz. glasses daily. Mentally decrease stress through daily relaxation. Lastly, for existing irritation and future health maintenance there is nothing better than Chiropractic care to maintain your health. Chiropractic adjustments add life to your years and years to your life.

Quote of the day: *"Don't worry about the world coming to an end today. It's already tomorrow in Australia."*—Charles Schultz

Back pain relief linked to combination of Chiropractic and exercise

Question: Is it a good idea to exercise while I have my back pain?

Answer: Every back condition is unique in its etiology. It depends on your degree of pain, location of pain, history of activity and many other factors. Exercise is exceptional for back conditions that can tolerate it. A recent British study published in *The American Medical Journal*, demonstrated that spinal manipulation was more effective when combined with exercise. It stated that the addition of exercise provided significant relief of symptoms and improvements in general health.

The type of exercise should be specific to your back condition. Many of the general spinal stretching exercises are similar to yoga postures and are very considerate of the delicate nature of its functions. Whether you have existing back pain or none at all, it is great preventative self-healing to do controlled spinal stretching on a daily basis. Most Chiropractors, Physical Therapists and many medical physicians are familiar with these stretches and can counsel you in starting a daily program. Making a New Year's resolution to start a spinal stretching program cannot only reduce pain, but can add life to your years.

Persistent pain or irritation while exercising are contraindications to performing the exercise and should be discontinued until you work with your Chiropractor to determine the cause of the discomfort.

Quote of the week: *"How beautiful a day can be when kindness touches it."*—G. Elliston

Beach chairs can irritate back conditions

Question: Every time I go the beach it seems I get low-back pain. Whether I sit in a beach chair or lye on the sand my muscles get sore and my back hurts. Is there a correct way to support my back at the beach?

Answer: Most beach chairs are made to be lightweight and are easily handled to gain access to the beach. There is not much ergonomic concern put into your typical inexpensive beach chair. Most people spend hours at the beach and may not get up at all or only get up to go into the water. Combine the extended time in an unsupportive chair with lengthy malposition of your spine and the result is going to be back discomfort. If you have a predisposition to back pain you are really asking for trouble. Always consider the three curves in your spine and their need to be supported. A flattening of any of the cures in your spine over taxes the adjacent muscles. You may feel comfortable with the hot sunshine and cool breeze on your body, but gravity will continue to push down on your spine. Many beach chairs conform your spine into a large "C". When you lean backward your unsupported mid-back falls into the thin fabric of the chair. The slanted angle of your body can unsuspectingly redistribute weight bearing to your lower spine. Initially, as the muscles settle into the unhealthy posture, you may not notice the shift of pressure. Over time the muscles will get tighter to protect you. By the time you get up and try to perform normal activity the over activated low back muscles can be eliciting a pain response.

The same is true for lying in the sand. Lying on your back or on your stomach for hours in the sand can transfer weight bearing to areas that normally don't receive stress.

The solution is to purchase a good low back supportive chair and be conscious of your posture prior to lying down. You can also support your spinal curves while lying on your back in the sand by pushing sand under your neck and low back where they form "C" curves.

Persistent low-back pains after the beach trip should be checked by a Chiropractor.

Quote of the week: *"The most important thing about goals is having one."*—Geoffrey F. Abert

Be aware of early warning signs of poor health

Question: How can I tell, as a layperson, that I may need to see a Chiropractor? What are the early warning signs?

Answer: Chiropractors detect and correct vertebral subluxations in the spine. Vertebral subluxations are misalignments of the vertebra secondary to the body's inability to compensate for any form of stress. The five components that create a vertebral subluxation complex include joint damage, nerve damage, tissue damage, muscle damage and overall heath degeneration. As long as you have a spine in this stressful world you can get vertebral subluxation complex (VSC).

Early warning signs of VSC that you can be conscious of include:

1. Having the heels of your shoes wear out unevenly.

2. Inability to take a deep breath.

3. Clicking in your jaw.

4. Excessive cracking in your neck, back, or other joints.

5. There is unequal movement when you turn your pelvis or neck side-to-side.

6. You are always tired.

7. You have poor concentration.

8. You have low resistance to disease.

9. Your foot or leg turns outward when you walk.

10. One leg is shorter than the other.

11. You have poor posture.

12. You consistently have sore, painful spots in your muscles, headaches, and backaches.

13. You feel constantly under stress, tense in your muscles and joints.

14. You just feel terrible in general.

If you've answered yes to one or any combination of these warning signs you should discuss it with a doctor of Chiropractic.

Chiropractors do not treat conditions; instead they correct the cause of disease or lack of body harmony.

Vertebral subluxations are very common and often painless. This is why Chiropractors suggest spinal check-ups for all members of the family. The correction of vertebral subluxations known as "an adjustment" is also gentle and painless in most cases.

Quote of the week: *"Do not worry about whether or not the sun will rise. Be prepared to enjoy it."*—Unknown

Bitter is better when it comes to fruits and vegetables

Question: You mentioned the term phytonutrients in you previous column. I am not sure what a phytonutrients, let alone what each vitamin and mineral does. Could you explain phytonutrient?

Answer: Phytonutrients are naturally occurring substances found in whole foods that may be more important to good nutrition than vitamins. In general, the more bitter the taste, the richer the food is with phytonutrients.

Recent research has discovered that phytonutrients can help prevent and treat cancer as well as other diseases. Their actions halt the production of cancer causing agents in the body, blocking activation of these chemicals, or suppressing the spread of cancer cells that already exist.

To get phytonutrients into your system you must first start eating you fruits and vegetables. The produce items researchers think are most capable of preventing cancer and other diseases, including heart disease, are green leafy vegetables, broccoli, Brussel spouts, cabbage, onions, citrus fruit (not citrus juice), grapes, red wine, green tea and others. The more bitter the better. To cut some of the bitterness, try adding sea salt, spices, small amounts of virgin olive oil, or butter.

The manufacturing process of these types of foods reduces their potency. Canned or frozen fruits or vegetables are never as nutrient rich as fresh. Growing your own or buying organic food will enhance your best potential to get the maximum phytonutrients from your food.

Additional phytonutrient-rich foods you could include in your diet are zucchini, other squashes, pumpkins, cucumbers, and melons, along with almonds and many types of beans. Pickling preserves phytonutrients in foods also.

Quote of the Week: *"We don't need more strength or more ability or greater opportunity. What we need is to use what we have."*—Basil S. Walsh

Breast-feeding helps infant eczema

Question: I take my two infants, ages 2 ½ months and 13 months to a Chiropractor and it has helped with their colic but now I notice eczema starting on my younger child. What can I do to help this condition?

Answer: It's wonderful to hear of more and more parents reaching out for natural solutions and healing approaches for their children's health and well being. Your solution to your child's eczema is closer than you may expect. Breast-feeding your child is the best way to reduce not only eczema, but also gastrointestinal infections in newborns and infants. If you already are nursing you should make a careful evaluation of your own personal diet. Make sure you are eating natural wholesome foods that are low on the allergy profile.

An article in the *Journal of the American Medical Association* supports previous evidence indicating that breast-feeding minimizes a newborn's odds of gastrointestinal infection and eczema.

The study polled data on 16,491 women and their newborns. The women received either traditional infant feeding or more extensive education aimed at maximizing the duration of breastfeeding. Babies whose mother's received more intense education about breastfeeding were more likely to be exclusively breast-fed and breast-fed for longer duration compared with women who did not receive special support. Youngsters who were breast-fed for 12 months were 40-percent less likely to experience gastrointestinal tract infections and 46-percent less likely to develop a-topic eczema, compared with babies who were breast-fed for fewer months.

Breast-feeding coupled with Chiropractic adjustments of your children will enhance their immune system and maintain a strong resistance to invading organisms.

Quote of the week: *"Ingenuity, plus courage, plus work, equals miracles."*—Bob Richards

Breast-feeding is best for newborns

Question: I am considering breast-feeding my newborn and was interested in your opinion as a pediatric Chiropractor.

Answer: My opinion is an overwhelming yes to breast-feeding your newborn. There is no better food for your baby. Cow's milk is for calves and a mom's milk is for her baby. The colostrum produced in the mother's milk for the first 6 to 8 weeks after birth contains every element necessary for a perfect immune system.

Unfortunately a recent study released by the World Health Organization (WHO) indicates a vast majority of mothers fail to follow even the minimum recommendations regarding breast-feeding from the American Academy of Pediatrics.

Experts recommend that women feed their babies exclusively on breast milk—no juice, no formula, and no food—for a minimum of 6 months, followed by breast-feeding supplemented with other foods for up to 2 years. These recommendations are based on research which shows that breast-fed babies grow better without getting fat and are less prone to infections—and these benefits last throughout childhood.

It's inexpensive, convenient, and it's uniquely tailored to meet all of baby's nutrition needs for the first 6 months of life.

Quote of the week: *"Parenthood remains the greatest single preserve of the amateur."*—Alvin Foffler

Cause of fatigue may be self evident

Question: I am 35-years-old and should be at the peak of my life as far as my energy levels, yet I am tired all the time. I have had all kinds of tests and none of them are positive. Could you give me a potential reason for this constant fatigue?

Answer: Fighting fatigue is the number one medical complaint by women in their 20s and 30s. The "fatigue syndrome" envelops millions of women yearly in both allopathic and natural healing circles. Medical physician Donnica L. Moore, president of Saphire Women's Health Group in Branchburg, NJ, believes that the prominent causes are sleep deprivation (most women in their 20s and 30s get under seven hours per night) and pregnancy. Other causes could be anemia, hypothyroidism hypoadrenia, and depression, over-or-under exercising, stress and the side effects of drugs including herbal supplements, anti-depressants and cold medicines.

One solution is to take on the problem as your own responsibility. Organize your activities; diet, habits, exercise routines, job functions and causes of stress by writing them down. As you write them take time to sense which activities hold a strong energy charge for you. For example: If writing chocolate down as a potential personal conflict makes you irritable it may be a source of concern. Prioritize those high-energy functions in order of their influence on your life. There may be people in your life that deplete your energy by being around them. Prioritize the people that squeeze energy from your life on a daily basis.

Once your lists are compiled decide on which items you can live without or avoid, starting from the most highly charged to the least charged. Your condition may not be physiologically discernable through medical testing because it may be a routine daily life exposure. You may be the only one to truly know your answer. Check your living environments, home, auto, office, etc. Exposure to mold, toxin, and allergens can deplete energy and fatigue the body.

Most importantly have your spine checked by a Chiropractor for neurological integrity. The nervous system is directly responsible for functions of energy. There are major traumas due to serious accidents and minor spinal malfunctions that occur in the normal course of daily living called vertebral subluxation. Severe traumas may cause immediate nerve irritation. However, the daily routine irritations more subtly exert pressure that slowly interferes with your nerves normal energy flow. While subluxations can result in pain, quite often they do not and if left uncorrected over a period of time, they can disrupt your nervous systems' normal function of relaying vital nerve impulses to essential body parts for energy.

Analyze your life and where your fatigue may be emanating from. Remove those interferences that you can control. See your Chiropractor for neurological fitness.

Quote of the week: *"I like long walks, especially when they are taken by people who annoy me."*—Fred Allan

Chiropractic can help you prevent the flu this winter

Question: Is there anything a Chiropractor can do to help me and my family prevent getting the flu this winter?

Answer: You can help yourself and family prevent the flu more than any one else. All the common sense rules your mother and her mother gave you still stand true. Here are a few important ones:

1. Wash your hands frequently with soap and hot water, rubbing vigorously for about 30 seconds.

2. Avoid touching your face, as germs on your hand may infect you through the eyes, nose and mouth.

3. Cough and sneeze into your elbow—not your hand—so that you do not spread germs if you are unable to wash immediately.

4. Get at least 7-hours of sleep a night (more for children)

5. Eat a varied and balanced diet that emphasizes plant foods, including whole grains, fruits and vegetables.

6. Avoid dairy products which are mucous forming and highly allergenic.

7. Drink at least six 12-ounce glasses of water a day to flush your system.

8. Exercise and sweat it out—it is shown to detoxify the body and boost the immune system.

Taking care of yourself is essential to a quick and healthy recovery. The most important rule is to get to your Chiropractor as soon as possible, after even the mildest of first signs or symptoms of a cold. The Chiropractic adjustment is exceptional in elevating the immune system. By balancing the nervous system the organs and glands responsible for fighting bacteria and viruses function to their highest potential and can fight against invading organisms.

People who are run down, overworked, and not getting proper rest or proper nutrition, are at a higher risk to invite disease and illness. Take care of yourself, use common sense, and see your Chiropractor and you will minimize the chance of getting the flu this winter.

Quote of the week: *"To disbelieve is easy; to scoff is simple; to have faith is harder."*—Louis L'Amour

Chiropractic, diet, and exercise assist blood pressure conditions

Question: Can Chiropractic help with high blood pressure?
Answer: The causes of hypertension (high blood pressure) are numerous. The correction or reduction of hypertension are also numerous. Modern medications have successfully treated blood pressure conditions for many years and are always improving. The natural methods of curbing a continually high and or dangerous blood pressure condition include Chiropractic, proper dietary habits, and moderate exercise.

Chiropractors adjust the vertebra of the spine to maintain a balance to the nervous system. The nerves enervating organs such as the adrenal glands and heart muscles must be functioning correctly for appropriate blood pressure to be regulated. Nutritional intake must include a healthy balance of fruit, vegetables and fiber along with fresh water, and healthy fats. That's right, healthy fats. Omega three fatty acids have clinically been shown to reduce cholesterol and unhealthy fats. Omega three fatty acids come from cold-water fish oils such as cod and salmon.

Moderate exercise is suggested, but a heart-rate monitor should be worn as a preventive measure. These monitors will notify you when you are outside your target heart range by beeping or flashing. Many heart attacks occurring during exercise are outside the target heart range. Consistent motion to all joints on a daily basis influences circulation to increase, which assists blood pressure.

Unmanaged stress on a mental or emotional level will affect blood pressure adversely. Unresolved issues that cause anxiety affect our blood pressure and should be attended to as a total well-rounded management of a hypertensive condition.

Some hypertensive conditions are genetically bound and even in these conditions utilizing the basic principals in this column will help.

Quote of the week: *"There is only one journey—going inside your-self."*—Rainer Maria Rilke

Chiropractic helps children

Question: Does Chiropractic help children and is it safe for them?

Answer: I am a pediatric-based Chiropractor and after 23-years of practice I am still amazed that the public is uninformed about the amazing success of Chiropractic with children. Children respond faster and more efficiently than adults. They have not established an over abundance of stress comparable to an adult. Stress and an over taxing of our nervous systems comes in many forms including mental, chemical, physical, family, relationships, jobs etc. Children are too young to have all of these complications and compiled stressors. Finding their irritations and causes of vertebral subluxations (interference to nerve supply due to vertebra moving out of their normal position) is easier because there are not layers of other problems covering the primary irritation. Vertebral subluxations in children are more cause and effect and once corrected respond with an immediate change or improved sense of well-being. Most of our children patients ask their parents to get adjusted and love coming to us because they know how much better they feel and they would rather get adjusted than take medications. Children have a special sense of what is safe and good and when they express a true attraction to a good cause a parent should not ignore them, just as when they sense that something is not safe.

Mounting scientific evidence suggests that Chiropractic care can be a natural management option for children suffering from such common conditions as otitis media (middle ear infection), colic, nocturnal enuresis (bedwetting), asthma, neurological disorders (such as epilepsy, autism, and attention deficit/hyperactivity disorder), headache, and many others.

The medical community is finally opening their eyes and letting go of their egos with the realization that there is significant benefit in working with Chiropractors to allow their pediatric patients every option in getting healthier naturally. Chiropractic is not the cure all for every ailment limiting a child's health but it is an excellent and safe way to get your child's general health condition evaluated.

Quote of the week: *"Love is what we were born with. Fear is what we learned here."*—Marianne Willamson

Chiropractic is a family affair

Question: I recently met a friend of mine who told me she takes her entire family to the Chiropractor. Originally, I knew she was going because of headaches and sinus conditions, which she said, were totally better. My question is how can Chiropractic be important to all members of the family?

Answer: One of the greatest healing capabilities enhanced by Chiropractic is the immune system function. All members of a family need a maximized immune function to fight illness and disease. Many people associate Chiropractic with neck pain, low-back pain, and musculoskeletal problem, when in actuality these are only secondary symptoms of malfunctions or misalignments of the spinal column called "vertebral subluxations". These vertebral subluxations can impinge nerves and disrupt their natural flow of energy to whatever cell, tissue or organ they enervate.

It is a misconception that you must have pain to have a need for a Chiropractor. Chiropractors can detect vertebral subluxations prior to a pain response as a preventative measure. Many patients have masked their conditions with drugs or been in denial of their pain for so long they can't even decipher its origin, even if it is a problem. Although vertebral subluxations often cause pain, there are many times they don't. This means that you or a member of you family could be subluxated and not even know it! That's why Chiropractic adjustments can benefit the entire family, from grandchildren to grandparents. At all stages of life, we each need our full natural flow of nerve energy (our "life force") to maintain optimum health and be free from pain, illness and disease.

Newborns get adjusted, too, because birth trauma and the delivery can cause a child's first subluxation even in a healthy natural childbirth. Children in general, respond exceptionally to gentle Chiropractic care because their conditions haven't been as patterned and buried for as long as most adults.

There's nothing that can stress a family more then ill health and disease. When one family member is not well, it affects the whole family. That's why we encourage our patients to make Chiropractic care a family affair.

Chiropractic is based on the principal that our natural state of health and well being is maintained by an "innate intelligence" flowing throughout nerves to all parts of our body. Chiropractic simply helps to keep this miraculous life force flowing freely by correcting "vertebral subluxations" (spinal misalignments) that interfere with vital verve energy impulses. Chiropractic is the world's leading natural care profession. Why don't you make your family a Chiropractic family?

Quote of the week: *"Tell me, I'll forget. Show me, I may remember. But involve me, and I'll understand."*—Chinese Proverb

Chiropractic is a mainstream healing profession

Question: I am a college student and I am considering Chiropractic as my career. My concern is whether Chiropractic has become mainstream or is just an alternative profession. My question is whether the Chiropractic profession is going to be accepted by the insurance industry in the future the same way the medical profession is accepted?

Answer: I can tell you are a good student already. You are looking into the future and gauging your opportunity and stability on facts. Chiropractic is the largest natural healing profession in the world. We started from humbled and contentious beginnings to its current state of mainstream healthcare providers. Chiropractic has improved its educational and licensing systems substantially giving it an increase in public credibility and improving its market share. The public utilizes Chiropractic largely for spinal pain syndromes and has a remarkable high patient satisfaction rate. The greatest inroads are in the private and public health care financing systems and are increasingly viewed as an effective specialty by many in the medical field.

Much of the positive evolution of Chiropractic can be ascribed to a quarter-century long research effort focused on the core Chiropractic procedure of spinal manipulation (adjustment). This effort has helped bring spinal manipulation out of the investigational category to become one of the most studied forms of conservative treatment for spinal pain.

I believe Chiropractic will be integrated into all health-care systems in the near future. Patient demand and patient satisfaction is higher now than ever. People are sick and tired of being sick and tired and Chiropractic is supplying a solution.

I hope your motivation to be a Chiropractor is not generated by money alone. I guarantee you will not survive long in a healing art such as Chiropractic if that is your priority. A great mentor taught me to serve for the sake of serving, give for the sake of giving and love for the sake of loving.

Quote of the week: *"You have reached the pinnacle of success as soon as you become uninterested in money, compliments, or publicity."*—O.A. Battista

Chiropractic is recognized around the world

Question: Is Chiropractic recognized in other countries?

Answer: Chiropractic is recognized worldwide. Third world countries as well as almost every country in the world have either practicing Chiropractors or have had exposure to Chiropractic science art and philosophy. Chiropractic remains the largest natural alternative healing art in the planet. Many believe that the Chiropractic philosophy of allowing the body to heal itself through a balanced nervous system and appropriate diet and exercise is overwhelmingly becoming the mainstream consciousness of the populace everywhere. I believe Chiropractic and natural healing will someday become the mainstream primary treatment of healthcare with medicine and surgery becoming the secondary and tertiary means of care only after the body looses its ability to correct itself.

In 2005 the first Chiropractic clinic opened in China. There are two major international Chiropractic associations and each country acknowledging Chiropractic has representatives as members. Princess Diane was influential in starting the first Chiropractic educational institutions in Great Britain just prior to her untimely death. Australia is a major proponent of Chiropractic and Chiropractic education with at least two colleges presently and more to follow. Canada has a strong Chiropractic community and mentality and it has been part of their culture and intertwined in society almost as long as in the United States since its discovery in 1885 by Dr. D. D. Palmer.

Foreign ambassador teams of "good will," commit and volunteer as Chiropractors abroad, to travel across the globe, spreading the art, philosophy and science of Chiropractic. These dedicated professionals give their personal time to adjust needy families in desperate and even dangerous regions of the world.

Chiropractic is recognized by even the earliest civilizations, including the Egyptians who noted the spine and its orientation to functions in the body on their hieroglyphic tablets written on stone. In fact, the name Chiropractic comes from the Greek term "Chiro"—Hand and "Practic"—The Practic Of, meaning the practice of placing the hands on the body for healing.

Quote of the week: *"There is nothing we cannot live down, rise above, and overcome."*—Ella Wheeler Wilcox

Chiropractors become unified

Question: Are there different types of Chiropractors and what is the difference between a straight and a mixer?

Answer: Chiropractors are very unique in that each Doctor of Chiropractic can choose from numerous clinical procedures and approaches to brand their particular style. In this sense Chiropractors are very different. Philosophically most Chiropractors share one primary dogma that keeps them unified. This major premise is that by removing the vertebral subluxation complex, (abhorrent neurological function, secondary to vertebral misalignment), the innate intelligence that heals the body can be released to return the body to homeostasis. The same intelligence that creates the body heals the body and its conduit of communication is through the nervous system. No other profession can specifically locate and correct vertebral subluxations. The unifying bond between all Chiropractors is their universal acceptance of the vertebral subluxation complex.

Straight or mixer Chiropractor are archaic terms. There are Chiropractors that choose to be called straight due to their rigid belief system in their approach to managing the vertebral subluxation. The mixer was considered any treatment outside the straight belief system. Chiropractic has evolved over its 100-plus years of existence. New ideas and techniques in approaching this vertebral subluxation complex (VSC) has improved and enhanced treatment. The original techniques are still very effective but there are advantages to the new techniques also.

The Chiropractors are unifying to present one voice for Chiropractic to the public. The many different Chiropractic organizations are attempting to move towards a unified front regarding laws that will help patients get timely appropriate care. It is an exciting time for the profession of Chiropractic, Chiropractors and their patients.

You can support your Chiropractor by registering to vote an asking him or her which politicians represent the right choices to benefit you and your care.

Quote of the week: *"The greatest thing in this world is not so much where we are, but in what direction we are moving."*—O. W. Holmes

Chiropractors hold the key to anti-aging

Question: Is it true that getting Chiropractic treatments can have an anti-aging affect?

Answer: Americans spend billions of dollars annually on products services and procedures to make themselves look and feel younger. The true answer to feeling and looking better is within you. Chiropractors are the ultimate guide to leading you to a life full of health and youthfulness. In a way Chiropractors are orthodontists of the spine. But, a crooked spine is much more detrimental to your health than crooked teeth.

Orthodontists put braces on teeth and adjust them regularly. Chiropractors don't use braces, but they make adjustments in a different way. These adjustments must be made regularly to get the full effect, since muscles and ligaments continue to pull the spine out of alignment when irritated. A Chiropractic adjustment corrects postural deviations in the spine which helps maintain a healthy nervous system which in turn helps all the other organs and systems in the body to remain healthy and viable.

Nutritional counseling on eating healthy can restore dying or stressed tissue. The aging process can be accelerated because of toxins in our body as well as a lack of specific nutrients. Chiropractors are positioned to give advice on proper eating habits as well as nutrition.

Diet, exercise, attitude, postural habits and ergonomics are all areas that Chiropractors teach their patients in educational classes and during treatments. You don't have to spend billions of dollars to stay young, just listen to your Chiropractor and believe in yourself.

Quote of the week: *"Though we travel the world over to find the beautiful, we must carry it with us or we find it not"*—Ralph Waldo Emerson

Chiropractors take aim at educating the public

Question: Why do Chiropractors have booths in the mall or at fairs? Why is it necessary for them to publicly advertise?

Answer: Some Chiropractors do utilize areas of high traffic to get direct one on one contact with the public. Chiropractors recognize that many people have never used their services nor understand what Chiropractors do. Advertising in newspapers, on radio, or even on television is pricey and may not be cost effective. Chiropractic is still considered an alternative health-care by many even though its has entered the mainstream of primary care providers. Because of all these factors many Chiropractors choose to take their message to the public rather than wait for the patient to walk in their door. Education of the public assists the patient in understanding that waiting for symptoms or temporarily managing pain is like putting a band aide on your health concern. Chiropractic attempts to find the cause of your condition permanently correct it and then educate the patient on how to prevent it from returning. Chiropractic teaches preventative maintenance and the management of healthy people as opposed to waiting for symptoms or sickness to come and go.

The challenge for today's Chiropractor is to educate the human being that health is a combination of the chemical, mental, spiritual and physical body and its ability to interact with its ever-changing environment. If stress could be piled high like a mountain, each component of the human being can contribute to the overall mass. Chiropractors remove the main stressors in your nervous system, which then allows all the other components to function better or to allow the individual to focus attention to the other causes of their stress.

Chiropractors attempt to stimulate this message one on one because it is an alternative to the western way of thinking. We call it a paradigm shift in consciousness. When making your choice as to which doctor or Chiropractor you would choose to administer your health care it makes a lot of sense to meet them and determine if you like them before making such an important decision. This seems more realistic than randomly choosing from an advertisement or the phone book.

Quote of the week: *"Act locally, think globally."*—Rene Dubos

Combined stretching and strengthening best management for low back

Question: What is the best method of maintaining my low back on my own to avoid pain and re-injury?

Answer: Combining stretching and strengthening along with cardiovascular routines for stamina, function to minimize low back pain and injuries.

Personalizing your conditioning workouts to your back condition and your goals is also essential to maintenance of a healthy spine. Runners should do more lower-extremity stretching and "cardio" workouts where as a swimmer would do more upper-extremity and possibly strengthening activities. A proper warm up and cool down prior to and following exercise is mandatory to reduce injury possibilities. I suggest all joints be stretched in a controlled environment, no matter what your sport preference is. A brief "cardio" warm up is always a good idea to get circulation to the body and engage the heart rate to increase in preparation for increased activity.

Always keep a good conscious focus on your body and spinal posture when exercising. Keep the curves of the spine in balance and maintain a straight spine whenever possible. Use your larger stronger muscles such as the gluteals in the buttocks and quadriceps in the front of the legs whenever possible.

Any continuous irritation or pain should be communicated to your Chiropractor to check for asymmetries or imbalances in your structure. Taking responsibility for your own health by maintaining your spine with stretching and strengthening will definitely keep your doctor bills down and enhance your quality of life.

Quote of the week: *"There is no exercise better for the heart than reaching down and lifting people up."*—John Andrew Holmes

Conquer your accident fears

Question: Is it normal to be scared to drive after an accident? How long should a fear like last and why do I feel my pains when even considering driving?

Answer: The brain is similar to a computer and it will continually play back input such as traumas or dramatic incidents in our lives. The initial interruption in the neurological processing can leave a strong imprint in thinking and normal response to similar situations can be altered. The nervous system will retrieve information most appropriate to every situation similar to the original trauma. An example of this, as in your case, would be a person getting into an automobile accident and traumatizing their head and neck in the accident as the vehicle ran into a tree. Months or even years later a person could have a repetitive loop played in the mind that every time they see a tree they get neck pain and headaches. The person may not have any idea why and consciously never remember the tree from the accident. This type of retracing of the brain has been labeled an engram in some psychological circles. We can develop these fears based on early life traumatic experiences and carry them around forever like bad luggage.

The brain is not the only area that continually reprints these micro and macro traumas. Our physical and emotional reactions become behaviorally patterned as well. Did you ever wonder why certain pains or emotions are elicited every time you are exposed to some person or event? We unfortunately feed our fears and engrams without even realizing it. A challenging factor for Chiropractors, and healers in general, is deciphering between what is a conditioned response to something that doesn't exist anymore and what is happening in present time existence. Receiving treatment immediately after any trauma is prudent to return normal responses back to the nervous system. Movement to a damaged joint is essential to restoring the functional feedback to the brain. Chiropractic treatment is very familiar with the effect of conditioned response and understanding that returning the normal function back to all injured areas of the body as soon as possible will minimize both physical and mental dependency in the future. If you get in an accident get to your Chiropractor as soon as possible.

Quote of the week: *"Nothing in life is to be feared. It is only to be understood."*—Marie Curie

Discuss destructive health habit changes with your doctor

Question: I am concerned about my husband's self-destructive health habits. He smokes cigarettes all day and eats everything in sight. He is over weight and his breathing is labored. My question is why his doctors don't talk to him and tell him the danger he is in?

Answer: Half the deaths in the United States are due to self-destructive behaviors, like your husbands, including smoking and over eating. About 1.3 million people die each year from conditions that could have been prevented or delayed by healthier habits.

I don't know why your husband's doctors don't discuss his heath habits. A study at Case Western Reserve University studied patient satisfaction in discussing behavioral issues. Only 48-percent of the physicians discussed behavioral issues during office visits. Discussing diet, exercise, alcohol, drug use, and prevention of sexually transmitted diseases does not put off most physicians. The study indicated patient satisfaction was much higher for those patients whose doctors did discuss behavioral concerns.

I believe healing comes from inside out. All patients are inevitable responsible for their own decisions on their health behaviors. It is absolutely the treating doctors responsibility, whether a M.D., D.C., or D.O., etc. to alert and inform their patient of their potential self-damaging behaviors. The doctor can offer advice for counseling or alternatives to avoid the self-defeating actions.

Even with this knowledge and the potential for health improvement people still make their own decisions to stop faulty behaviors.

Your husband may need a greater motivational boost to make his decision to stop his self-destruction. Lead through example of your own integrity and keep improving yourself. Leave alternatives out for him to see or read. Talk to his physicians and request they speak to him about these behaviors.

Quote of the week: "*The seasons do not push one another; neither do clouds race the wind across the sky. All things happen in their own good time.*"—Dan Millman

Don't underestimate your brain

Question: How important is the brain in controlling my spine and back pains?

Answer: A brain by itself may not be impressive, especially with its gooey blob-like appearance. It is 85-percent water and looks like Jell-O. The great intellect Aristotle only believed that the brain existed to cool down the blood. The brain does receive 20-percent of the body's blood supply, but the brain can cool the blood solely through rational thought.

We have technologically advanced ourselves as a species, yet we still do not totally understand the entire potential capacity of our brains. We do know this; it is compact and weighs about 3 pounds, it has efficient power consumption (equivalent to a 20-watt light bulb), has massive storage capacity (100 trillion bits of information), and is still more efficient than any computer. A fully developed human brain contains 100 billion neurons (nerve cells) as opposed to the lowly worm's 23. The number of neurons, however, is not as important for intelligence and healing as the connections between them. They communicate via neurotransmitters or chemical messengers. When one neuron fires off a message, it is received in one of thousands of receptor sites in another neuron, which stops it or sends it on. When too many neuron transmissions are sent or not sent the result is excess activity to a tissue, organ, or gland etc. or insufficient activity. A classic example in your back would be; a stressful day that caused tension and anxiety induced a constant tightness in your neck and shoulder muscles. While you were stressing out, neurons were transmitting excessively to the involved muscles which in turn attached to vertebra and caused them to misalign (subluxate) resulting in a symptom of pain or any sensory or motor dysfunction. This typical scenario demonstrates how abhorrent thought process can excite or diminish the brain's transmissions to the rest of the nervous system and therefore affect any function in the body. We only use about half our brain so don't underestimate its potential.

Quote of the week: *"A conclusion is a place where you got tired of thinking."*—Arthur Bloch

Drug ads directed to consumer, not physicians

Question: I live in a retirement community and it seems everyone is taking drugs for their back conditions. Why is there such an overabundance of drug use, especially anti-inflammatories, for people with back pain and arthritis?

Answer: The answer is direct-to-consumer drug advertising by pharmaceutical companies. The drug industry is the most influential lobbying body and marketing mastermind in the country. Their mass media advertisements create illusions about the healing ability found in their pills. Drug manufacturers are getting away with misleading and potentially dangerous communications to the public about their super drugs, yet they are being allowed to delete vital information regarding side effects and overuse. Their brainwashing of the public has caused consumers to demand drugs such as Cox-2 inhibitors, steroidal and non-steroidal anti-inflammatory drugs targeted at back pain and rheumatoid arthritis.

The United States is the only English speaking country that allows drug companies to pitch their prescription drug products directly to patients. Ads are designed to encourage patients to request the advertised drug from physicians. This puts physicians in an uncomfortable predicament. They can review the patient's history to decide if the drug is appropriate and prescribe it. They can prescribe it against their better judgment or they can not prescribe it, possible damaging their doctor-patient relationship. I believe patients should educate themselves about any medication they may need prior to usage but they should respect their physician's professional advice regarding potential usage and its dangers. Hopefully this is why you have entered your physician's office in the first place.

Richard L. Kravitz, an MD from the University of California at Davis did a research study on drug ads, examining 320 print ads touting 101 drug brands. The ads were combined from 18 popular magazines published between 1989 and 1998 on an 11-point education scale (11 representing optimal educational quality), the average scored only 3.2 points. According to Kravitz et al, many ads failed to provide adequate information. Only 9 percent of the ads reported a drug's typical success rate.

Fewer than 30 percent of the drug companies mentioned that there were alternative treatments for the same condition. Only 36 percent told how the drug worked. And only 24 percent told consumers about potential lifestyle alterations that could improve the condition, with or without administration of the drug.

Medical physicians should start exerting pressure on the drug industries to incorporate more information about condition and treatments in its advertising. Physicians should also keep evidence based educational materials on hand to inform patients of pros and cons of various pharmaceuticals.

You the consumer should access all information of the medication, and not just go by the drug ad slanting its opinion toward the utilization of its product.

An excellent alternative to drug usage for rheumatoid arthritis and back pain is Chiropractic. Advise your friends, family and neighbors to consider Chiropractic first as a conservative, safe, painless alternative to medications for low-back and many arthritic conditions.

Quote of the week: *"Every situation properly perceived, becomes an opportunity."*—Helen Schucman

Early detection of postural changes in children allows proper growth

Question: I am concerned about my infant's spine growing straight. What can I do to make sure he develops properly?

Answer: As a parent, you can be extremely helpful in observing postural changes in your children. At birth, observation of symmetry of an infant's skull, pelvis and extremities can indicate potential growth and development problems.

There are basically four critical stages of weight bearing adjustment after birth that a parent should be aware of. The first stage is when the infant initially raises his/her own head (approximately 2-to 3-months of age) and starts to arch the neck in an attempt to develop its first curve in the cervical spine. Look for excessive lateral tilting to one side or responding to stimulus by always rotating or bending the head to the same side.

The second critical stage of weight bearing is crawling. The cross-crawl mechanism of moving opposite arms and legs forward and then backwards, is a vital developmental action of the brain in coordinating body movement. Greater than 80-percent of one side of your brain controls the opposite side of the body. The cross-crawl action of the baby develops brain-body coordination as well as stimulates growth of your child's nervous system. An improper cross-crawl mechanism in infants deters nervous system function, growth and coordination. Observer your infant for proper opposition movement, dragging of one or both legs, pulling with just upper or lower extremities. The problem may only be a pelvic or upper-back subluxation (misaligned vertebra creating nerve pressure) which can be corrected with Chiropractic care.

The third phase of weight bearing and postural change is at (3-to 6-months of age) when an infant begins to pull itself up and put weight onto legs and then their low back, creating the second lordotic curve.

Parents can observe for the same changes they would see in the cervical spine and a tendency to let all the weight go to one leg. You may notice he/she constantly falls to one side. Observe the crease created by the buttock while the baby lies on his/her stomach. Does it deviate dramatically to the left or right? This can indicate imbalance in the pelvic bones.

The fourth and final critical stage of weight bearing for an infant occurs when he/she starts to walk. An early stage of walking means falling often. This is part of learning. We don't just get on a bike and start to ride. Your child learns from each attempt they make. Do not assist your toddler, especially with walking devices. Once again, these interrupt brain to body coordination and may prematurely put weight bearing on hip, leg and low back joints. Be patient and observe for excessive falling to one side, toes pointing out (externally) or in (internally) on one or both sides, knees turned in or out. Also, observe for constant falling forward or backward. These could all indicate improper growth plate development, proprioceptive ability, or joint dysfunctions.

Once walking, the spine and weight bearing joints will grow in response to the stress put on them. Scoliosis (lateral curvature of the spine) can be observed by a parent by having their child bend at the waist letting their arms dangling in from of them. Observe from behind your child looking directly up the spine. Any dramatic asymmetries of large muscle bulked higher on either side could indicate scoliosis.

As the twig bends so does the tree. As the spine grows it will deviate around these imbalances and could create severe cosmetic as well as organic encroachment in the future.

The beauty of nature for children is that the body wants to grow straight and be healthy. Should some postural imbalances be detected, have your child checked by a heath professional preferably a Chiropractor that specializes in the spinal biomechanics. Many conditions do correct themselves but for the ones that don't, early detection and correction can prevent a lifetime of problems. Treatment for children is usually gentle and brief.

Quote of the Week: *"We cannot direct the wind...but we can adjust the sails."*—Unknown

Early to bed kids are healthier

Question: I have two elementary school-age children that want to stay up late, even on school nights. Is it true that staying up late at their ages is unhealthy and stressful? Please verify if this is true or not.

Answer: I emphasize with your predicament regarding late night bedtime for elementary school age children. I have two boys myself and must battle to get them to bed early every school night. The answer to this for your children and my children and every other parent that has the same concern is yes, early to bed children fair better emotionally and physiologically. A study done at Brown University Medical School gave 138 third grade girls stressful tasks during a few hours spent at their homes. The researchers measured initial levels of the stress hormone cortisol in saliva samples and rechecked cortisol after each task. The girls' weeknight bedtimes correlated with their stress hormone response. Those going to bed early released more cortisol after the first stressful experience, but compared with girls kept up past 9 p.m., their stress hormones declined more steeply during the next two tasks. Kids with later bed times, were more uncomfortable during the tasks than the children who got more sleep.

Prolonged output of cortisol can:

- raise blood pressure and heart rate,

- weaken immune response, so that colds and other viruses take hold more easily, and

- make it harder to concentrate when challenged.

The findings apply to boys as well as girls. The study also found preliminary evidence of nervous system changes in sleep-deprived children. Children's sleep needs vary and the majority can handle mild degrees of sleep depravations, but some do just terribly.

It can sometimes be stressful just putting your children to bed at the appropriate time. I personally would rather deal with an upset child at bedtime than a cranky child in the morning, especially when attempting to meet deadlines as well as making sure the children eat a healthy breakfast.

I agree with you that a parent's responsibility is to get their child to bed at a reasonable time and to maintain a consistency in that time to reduce stress and maintain a healthy nervous system.

Quote of the week: *"Experience...is simply the name we give our mistakes."*—Oscar Wilde

Education is essential for healthy patient

Question: Why do Chiropractors persistently attempt to give their patients educational material about health and conditions?

Answer: It is true that many Chiropractors share the philosophy that an educated patient is a healthier patient. The main reason educational material regarding Chiropractic is disseminated to their patients is to create a paradigm shift in their belief system regarding how the body heals and what causes dysfunction in the their beings. Modifying a behavior is difficult enough in itself but modifying a belief system that has been instilled in a patient their entire life is even more challenging. The majority of first time Chiropractic patients enter the Chiropractor's office with a medical allopathic model. This belief system basically implies that we are not born healthy and must be dependent on drugs and external support to maintain a healthy lifestyle. The medical model also implies that we don't need to consider that we have a problem with our health until we have a symptom.

The Chiropractic philosophy teaches that we are born to be perfect and 100-percent of our potential should be maintained at all times. Life and healing comes from within, and ultimately the maintenance of health is superior to the treatment of disease. I personally believe in this so much that it makes up the mission statement on the back of my business card.

Transitioning a patient from allopathic to natural belief systems requires education and repetition of input. Brochures, videos, tapes, lectures and one-on-one descriptions support the patient in understanding more about the truths of health rather than be swayed by myths and lies. The bottom line is how a patient feels after treatment, not only in their initial stages of care, but also in the long term. A patient that understands they are equally as responsible for their own health as their Chiropractor will actively participate in a team effort to grow their health to its maximum potential. Chiropractic, along with proper diet, exercise, mental-stress balancing, and a proper philosophical mindset equals a happy healthy person.

Quote of the week: *"The man who cannot believe in himself cannot believe in anything else."*—Roy L. Smith

Environment can influence health

Question: I noticed that when I am on vacation, away from my home or from my office, my health improves, including my neck pain. Can being in the environment of my home or office be causing my neck pain?

Answer: Environmental influences on an individual's health is very real. At home you may be exposed to any variety of airborne toxins or natural allergins from the vegetation around you. Your bed or couch that you use to sleep in or watch TV may be a poor form of posture support. At work there are potential irritants to your health from carbon products, improperly positioned computer work stations, bending of the head for extended phone conversation, and many many more. Besides objects and chemical irritants in your environment there can be another person in your space that creates stress for you.

Any and all the above potential environmental stressors can trigger physical response from the body by way of the nervous system. Overloads of stress by steady exposure to your toxic environment results in symptoms. Many people feel their symptoms in their neck or develop headaches. Others bear their stress in their stomachs or bowels, therefore the incredible high incidence of irritable bowel syndrome and associated conditions. Like yourself, it isn't until we are removed from the stressors that we realize our symptoms are normal responses to the overload of those daily exposures whether small or large. You are fortunate to identify that you feel better when away from your environment. Your next challenge is to identify what or who is creating an unhealthy environment and create an approach to conquer these irritants. Checklists of the contents of each room and how they are utilized is a good start. Next, take a conscious emotional evaluation of how you feel when in the presence of the people you suspect are irritating you. Obviously you can't always remove these people from your life, but you can express your concern and hopefully restore a healthy relationship.

Should your condition persist, try consulting your Chiropractor to see if he can assist you in determining the source of your stress.

Quote of the week: *"A moment's insight is sometimes worth a life's experience."*—Oliver Wendell Holmes

Everyone gets vertebral subluxations

Question: It seems that everyone I know now goes to a Chiropractor. They all tell me their Chiropractors say they have subluxations. Is it true that everyone gets vertebral subluxations?

Answer: Vertebral subluxations exist in epidemic proportions in modern day society. No one is immune to neurological stress or any stress for that matter. Whoever created us, designed us to be perfectly self-healing organisms. If we didn't keep messing with the natural systems we were given we wouldn't have any disease or illness. The reality is that life is stressful for everyone. Some stress is good, like happy stress such as winning money and some stress is difficult, like loosing a loved one. An inability to adapt to the stress in our own personal environment is a reflected as neurological distress.

Spinal malfunction is a common health problem that can be caused by neurological distress, long periods of sitting, standing, bending, improper lifting, overexertion, and many activities we consider normal. Fortunately the body and nervous system can correct many of these spinal problems on its own. Yet, the only way to deal with the vertebral subluxation complex (VSC) is by specific spinal adjustments to improve bio-mechanical function and remove nerve system interference.

Chiropractors themselves get adjustments on a regular basis. I check my own children weekly and my associate and I check each other weekly, for VSC. Most of the time we all require adjustments to keep our maximal potential at peak performance. We do not live with bubbles around us warding off anything that could irritate or subluxate us. The truth is we all do have VSC and we all should get checked by a Chiropractor on a regular basis. There is only one way to rid yourself of VSC and that is by a Chiropractor. Adjusting vertebral subluxations is what defines the Chiropractic profession and distinguishes it from all other healing arts. Chiropractic remains the largest alternative healing art in the world and it does so do to its simplistic philosophy. The body has the ability to heal itself and will do so when it's natural channels are free to function. Correction of VSC allows the body to heal itself.

Quote of the week: *"If people never did silly things, nothing intelligent would ever get done."*—L. Wittgenstein

Excess video-game playing can injure wrists

Question: Can my son develop carpal-tunnel syndrome from playing video games all the time?

Answer: Any repetitive motion, consistently performed over a long period of time, taxes the ligaments and tendons of that joint.

I have first hand observed children and adults play these games for hours and days on end. I have a personal vendetta to destroy all Gameboys and video games, so I will try to be objective as possible. When hours of play turns into days, weeks, months and even years, I believe it is no longer a fad but an addiction and in some cases an obsession. Our children are members of the most obese generation in the history of mankind and if you don't think that the video industry and the enormous hours kids play these machines are directly affecting a new culture then you must be very naïve or blind. I know every parent is cheering for me now. My own children want to lynch me.

Getting back to the subject at hand, the answer to whether or not all this video-game hyper control knob banging contributes to wrist problems is obvious. Yes, it does irritate fingers, hands wrists and elbows not to mention warp the mind and have kids live in a fantasy world. These conditions can worsen if not attended to, including the warped mind. Symptoms from, lets call it, "controller abuse" can range from loss of strength, numbness, pain and loss of motion in any or all of the regions mentioned above.

My advice is to minimize the time your child wastes on video games and get him outside to exercise. Take a nice hike in the woods or to the beach and remind him what nature is like. How about read a book? Use the gameboy or video as a treat only. If your child's wrist still hurts then consider taking him to a Chiropractor. Chiropractors specialize in correcting neurological interruption in the body. Carpal tunnel is just one of many potential problems he may have. Dramatically reducing his control banging time should allow his condition to improve. If not, call your Chiropractor, but leave the Gameboy at home.

Quote of the week: *"When you don't have a grip on life, it will definitely get a grip on you."*—Jewel Diamond-Taylor

Excessive TV watching can be hazardous to a child's health

Question: I am trying to limit the amount of time my two children watch TV. I know it is bad for their health but would like a professional health care provider to acknowledge how it effects their health. Can you please explain to my kids and me why a lot of TV is unhealthy?

Answer: Television is absolutely hazardous to anyone's health, especially when it is utilized for mindless loss of valuable time. For children in today's society TV is one of the greatest downfalls to the health of our future generations. The average 6-to 11-year-old child watches about 24-hours of TV per week. The problem is that the more they watch in their younger years, the more likely they are to become overweight in their teen years. Increased TV time is directly proportional to increased snack and eating time as well as decreased exercise time. Exercise for a 6-to 11-year-old is crucial at this time for muscle and bone development along with co-ordination skills. The incidence of obesity increases by 2 percent for every hour of TV viewed by 12- to 17-year-olds. Twenty percent of teens who watch more then 5 hours of TV a day are obese while only 10 percent of teens who watch for an hour or less have a weight problem.

As a pediatric Chiropractor I am concerned about the lost mental capacity and lost life experience but more importantly the effect of obesity on children in developmental stages. Additional weight in the stomach exaggerates developing spinal curves while putting excess stress on spinal discs as well as other weight bearing joints. A healthy spine has a healthy support system, mainly muscles in the stomach, back and legs. If you want to minimize the risk of a backache or the possibility of scoliosis for your child, have them avoid being overweight and keep their supporting muscles, especially their abdominal muscles strong.

There is a definite relationship between poor health and excessive TV. Read a book, play outside, enjoy nature and be creative for the sake of a healthy body.

Quote of the week: *"Image creates desire. You will what you imagine."*—J. F. Gallimore

Exercise best therapy for chronic fatigue

Question: I have been diagnosed with chronic-fatigue syndrome and nothing medicinally has helped. I am exhausted from being exhausted. Is there anything you could suggest to help me?

Answer: Research on chronic-fatigue syndrome indicates that behavior-based therapies, including exercise, may be among the most effective treatments.

A review was published in the *Journal of the American Medical Association* (JAMA) that indicates a potential source of the cause of the syndrome is psychological and behavioral therapy very advantageous. Dr. Anthony Komaroff a professor of medicine at Harvard University Medical School, says "It helps people cope, with the illness, but it's not curative. In order to come up with really good treatments, you need to understand more about causes."

Once given the misnomer "yuppie flu," chronic fatigue syndrome is a complex, hard-to-diagnose illness. It involves persistent, debilitating fatigue that renders many patients bedridden. Any variety of other symptoms are also usually present, including memory problems, depression and flu-like signs such as fever, chills, and joint pain.

Abnormalities in the body's disease-fighting immune system have been found in many patients, and some researchers think viruses or defects in the body's ability to regulate blood pressure can trigger the disease. The diagnosis is generally made by excluding other illnesses.

The JAMA study discussed counseling in coping strategies such as stress management and a program of gradually increasing exercise showed the most promising results.

My personal clinical experience with many chronic fatigue syndrome patients treated in our office is that they all respond with some degree of improvement with Chiropractic care. Those that learned to cope with stress and perform regular exercise regimes while under care did even better symptomatically.

Quote of the week: *"You are a success when you have made friends with your past, are focused on the present, and are optimistic about your future."*—Zig Ziglar

Explain your pain

Question: Why don't most doctors relate to generalized pain? I feel when I tell my doctors that I have a pain all over he doesn't take me seriously. What can I do to explain my pain?

Answer: Ironically, generalized pain is one of the most common complaints to bring a patient into a doctor's office, yet can be the most difficult to diagnose and treat. Doctors can't measure pain objectively the way they can blood pressure or cholesterol levels. So when pain doesn't immediately respond to treatment, physicians and patients often accept it as just another symptom that has to be lived with.

Your concern is shared nationwide. A group of health-care organizations are now uniting to standardize a method to assess and treat pain. The new protocol gives the patients rights to allow their pain to be assessed and managed appropriately as well as documented.

All doctors and hospitals are now required to abide by these new protocols. You can help as a patient by first, not suffering in silence. Surveys have shown that many patients don't tell doctors or nurses about their pain for fear of being labeled cranky of difficult or because they assume that their discomfort will go away. In our office we have a large poster in the consultation room that reads, "I thought it would go away".

Pain is usually the last symptom to show up after a series of conditions or reactions occur improperly in the body. Pain is a protective mechanism of the body to let us know something is very wrong. Don't mask or hide your pain, rather understand it is a message from your body to seek help or make adjustments.

Secondly, if your current treatment isn't controlling your pain tell your medical doctor or your Chiropractor. Lastly, make yourself educated about your treatment. Ask questions; learn about your medications and their side effects. It is true that addiction can occur from painkillers but patients can also build a tolerance and loose the effect of the medication.

Consider alternatives other than drugs if they are not working. Chiropractic may be the solution you are looking for.

Quote of the week: *"Whether you think you can or think you can't, you are right."*—Henry Ford

Extra vertebra is a common anomaly

Question: My Chiropractor reviewed my X-rays and discovered that I have an extra vertebra in my low back. Does this mean I am a freak?

Answer: You may be a freak but it isn't because of your extra vertebra. Any change from normal anatomy is considered an anomaly. Approximately 7 percent of the population have anomalies in their spine. Many anomalies are seen as extra vertebra. It is most common to observe extra vertebra in the lower lumbar spine because during growth and development your sacral bone is segmented prior to fusing into one solid mass. The lumbar vertebra above the sacrum look very similar to the sacral segments and the upper segment may not fuse entirely allowing it to create a rudimentary disc between the 5th lumbar and sacrum. In some cases this disc is functional and will develop identically to a lumbar vertebra with nerve supply to the lower torso. Most lumbarization is benign to the body and is asymptomatic as far as spinal function. Many patients demonstrate longer torsos or spines with extra vertebra, and many may be even more flexible in their pelvic region.

When there is one anomaly there is usually additional ones in that persons anatomy. The boney processes that extend from the vertebra are commonly misshapen, by being too long or too short compared to normal symmetrical processes. One could argue that we are all freaks since no human body is designed absolutely perfect and symmetrical. Our leg lengths are usually slightly altered and digits of the anatomy not exactly the same from extremity to extremity.

The cause of these anatomical phenomena is genetic. You could blame your parents or any member of your family tree. Someone messed with the DNA and mixed up some unusual combination of dominant and recessive genes to make you so unique. You are not a freak; you are special and one of a kind.

Quote of the week: *"The end of every maker is himself."*—St. Thomas Aquinas

Fibromyalgia linked to fatigue syndrome

Question: I have fibromyalgia and still don't understand what causes it. What does cause it and why is there so much confusion over it.

Answer: Fibromyalgia is a mysterious illness with a bad reputation. The symptoms range from inexplicable pain, stiffness, fatigue to full body joint ache. Most patients in the past were told that they were stressed out, depressed or it was psychosomatic. There is such an abundance of these combined symptoms that much attention has been focused on this syndrome. Researches and clinical data now imply that fibromyalgia is linked to chronic-fatigue syndrome and possible the after-effects of Lyme's disease.

Other theories contest that fibromyalgia can be due to decreased blood supply to the parts of the brain that process pain and twice the normal level of a brain chemical called "substance P" which helps the nervous system cells send pain messages to the brain. Another more radical theory contends that residual effects of antibiotic and vaccine treatments express themselves after years of dormancy.

The complaints are serious, from swelling, tingling, numbness, and stiffness in soft tissues (muscles, tendons, ligaments) to aching, throbbing pain that is worse in the morning, intensifies again at night and has been known to drive suffers to suicide. Fatigue is one of the most common complaints (reported in as many as 9-out-of-10 cases) caused perhaps by disturbances in the deep-sleep phase the body needs to get properly refreshed at night. Women get fibromyalgia seven times more than men do for some unknown reason.

There is no known cure for fibromyalgia. Many patients manage their pain with aerobic exercises such as cycling and jogging. Others feel stretching and yoga are effective. Many patients utilize massage and Chiropractic as their primary treatment.

Quote of the week: *"There are risks and costs to action. But they are far less than the long-range risks of comfortable inaction."*—President John F. Kennedy

Follow Mother Theresa's lead

Question: Many patients come in daily, disgusted with the state of human relations and their interactions with people on a daily basis. They have progressively been sharing with me that people are becoming mean and inconsiderate. They ask if I know why?

Answer: I would like to attend to this unfortunate but often asked question with a quote from Mother Theresa, "God does not command that we do great things, only little things with great love".

When we get overwhelmed with negative experiences we sometimes are consumed by negative thoughts. It takes great discipline to remove the onslaught of a series of unpleasant episodes. Forgiveness is essential and changing your perspective is even more beneficial. It is essential to discipline ourselves to focus on the "little things". The "things" that are good and positive. The general overwhelming state of affairs can appear grim at times but you can erase the displeasure by concentrating on the small stuff such as loved ones in your life. In any situation I first ask myself if my children's lives are endangered by the actions at hand. Second, I determine if my health or welfare is endangered. If no danger or health risk exists then it is just small and insignificant to me. You will find that 90 percent of the so-called "bad stuff" truly is insignificant.

Develop a "Teflon attitude" to verbal abuse and abhorrent behaviors of others. Lead through example. Reacting with anger, formulating retaliation or acting irreverently only hardens a bad situation. According to some patients there are plenty of "bad situations" to practice being "Teflon" to deflect.

Raise your standards and take control of yourself. Life is an ongoing learning experience. By meeting the challenge and overcoming adversity you will become empowered. Choose to be more caring and compassionate. You will be more powerful and happier in the end.

Quote of the week: *"A friend can tell you things you don't want to tell yourself."*—Frances Ward Weller

Forgiveness is healing

Question: Can there be a relationship between my headaches, ill health, and my inability to get over the separation from my significant other?

Answer: Loss of a loved one, whether it is due to death, divorce or permanent separation is considered by Dr. Hans Cele, an authority on stress research, to be one of the highest levels of stress on his charts. More than the stress of the initial shock of loss is the inability to forgive.

Forgiving all others is necessary as well as an effective purging to cleanse you for a renewed successful life. We don't have to like another person, persons or situation, just forgive them and let go of the mental chains that entrap us.

I have found in 24-years of practice, that mental and physical illnesses are inseparable. Your thoughts control your actions and therefore your eventual expression of life and health. We are all dealt some difficult hand to play in life. I find that those patients that accept their loss and forgive themselves, their situations and all people included, rebound and minimize any ill health effects. I find most suffering is self-induced. The fear of what the future will be like without the relationship they once had, creates illness. There is an acronym F.E.A.R. that stands for Future Events Appear Real. Focusing on non-existent future or the historic past disrupts our present time being consciousness leading to sickness.

It is imperative to live in the present and forgive. *Carpe Diem* (seize the moment) and you will see a transformation in your life and health.

Quote of the week: *"A journey of thousand miles begins with a single step."*—Lao Tzu

Give yourself the gift of Chiropractic

Question: What health-supportive gifts would you suggest for my family for the holidays?

Answer: There is no better gift for your health than the gift of Chiropractic. Remember, you are asking a Chiropractor. We inspire and motivate our active patients to consider the people in their lives that are less fortunate with their health. Many people suffer needlessly and could easily benefit from a painless Chiropractic adjustment. Most Chiropractors do not advertise, but depend on the direct referrals from their satisfied patients. Putting that much faith in the abilities of your own treatments means that it must be working. Our office and many other Chiropractic centers encourage patients with friends, family, neighbors or co-workers that are skeptical or frightened, to take advantage of a free consultation to learn for themselves exactly what we do. There is no obligation for these consultations. Once people realize that Chiropractic is based on natural functions and scientific facts they have less fear in considering this form of healthcare. Most people fear the unknown or rumors of false claims.

While you are shopping in the malls and retail stores across Ocean and Monmouth counties think of how your neck, back, shoulders, and legs feel as you are carrying all those heavy packages, getting in and out of vehicles, waiting in lines and stress over your finances. As wonderful as the spirit of the holidays can be uplifting and heartfelt, the reality is they are stressful and taxing on the mind and body. The perfect gift and solution to balance your holidays is a Chiropractic adjustment.

To all my readers, may your holidays be filled with love, joy, peace, health and happiness.

Quote of the week: *"The purpose of human life is to serve, and to show compassion and the will to help others."*—Albert Schweitzer

Grieving is normal and healthy

Question: I have been overwhelmed with grief from the results of the terrorist attacks on our nation. Watching TV, listening to the radio and always thinking of the victims and their families has me unable to function. What can I do to stop the grieving?

Answer: You are not alone, we are a nation of grieving souls. You are very normal and your grief is part of healing. It will get better for you and our nation. Keep talking to friends, neighbors and loved ones about your emotional upsets. Grieving with others allows you to confront your pain. Participating in candle light vigils, prayer and demonstrating your solidarity to this great nation will also help your healing process.

Physically avoid being dormant or stuck in front of your TV. Physical activity, exercise or even a walk along the beach or in the woods can ground your emotions. Remember to breathe and appreciate the beauty in your environment. Spend time with small children to remind yourself to laugh and be uninhibited.

Your brain is an organ just like your liver or kidney and it needs to rest occasionally. Grieving excessively can tax your brain and make you feel overwhelmed and fatigued. Don't stop grieving until you feel completely content you are done. Do take breaks and step away from the intensity to keep balance. Eat properly. Grieving can result in eating too much, too little or eating with a poor nutritious diet.

Get enough sleep and try to do a little relaxation prior to bed. Meditate, listen to comforting music or take a warm bath. Avoid watching TV right before bed because it leaves subliminal messages with you that can interrupt sleep.

Always remember to tell all your loved ones you love them. It is terrible that it takes a disaster to remind us of the important but simple daily measures we sometimes take for granted.

There is healing and comfort around the corner for you and America. We grow and heal in direct proportion to the catastrophic event that wounds us. Remember that we are wounded as a whole nation, but we will remain the most loving and caring people on this planet. The world is watching us to see how we heal. America has always been the leader in all worldly transformations.

I am confident we can teach the world how to heal, by our own unified efforts as a nation and God's protection. God Bless America.

Quote of the week: *"Healing in its fullest sense requires looking into our heart and expanding our awareness of who we are."*—Mitchell Gaynor

Head and facial injuries require immediate attention

Question: I was in a car accident 10 years ago. I damaged bones in my face and skull after hitting the windshield. I thought I was better after a few months but recently I am having sinus problems, headaches and visual changes. Is there a relationship between my old injuries and these conditions?

Answer: The body creates scar tissue, fibrotic tissue, and calcium repair within 48 hours of an injury. This healing mechanism is very normal and natural. The side effects of the laying down of healing tissues are loss of mobility and interruption of the function of adjacent healthy tissues.

Initially the injured tissues require immediate repair while overtime the accumulation of these thicker more dense healing elements can create problems.

In your specific condition the excess fibrotic tissue mass and calcified healed bones in your head and face may have developed slowly after the initial healing phase. The sinuses can be occluded or impinged, not allowing appropriate drainage. This can lead to facial pressure and headaches. Cranial sutures and structures move with respiration. Thickening of cranial bones and/or sutures disrupts normal expansion and contraction. These too can cause cranial pressure and headaches.

The answer to your question is, yes, it is very likely your former injury contributed to your present condition. The solution for anyone with a recent or past facial/cranial injury is to minimize the over production of the fibrotic tissue and induce motion into the fixed joints of the face and skull. This can be accomplished with massage and cranial bone balancing techniques. Many massage therapists and Chiropractors are trained in these techniques and could possibly help you.

Quote of the week: *"The past gives us experience and memories, the present gives us challenges and opportunities, the future gives us vision and hope."*—William Arthur Ward

High heels are a potential hazard

Question: I wear high heels and have been told they are bad for my feet and back. I prefer the way I look with heels. Is it bad to wear high heels?

Answer: Many women patients of ours have decided to wear more comfortable shoes for daily business and at home use. Besides feeling safer, they wear them because it's healthier.

High heels force an unnatural posture upon the foot and low back. High heels shorten the muscles of the calves and compromise this muscle group with extended wear. These types of footwear put all the weight forward on the balls of the feet (metatarsals), which is naturally intended to be redistributed equally across the entire foot.

I am always concerned about long term high heel utilization when considering the Chiropractic model of spinal balance. High heels shove the pelvis forward stressing the lower back, forcing it into an unnatural, dangerously misaligned curve. It is very common to observe chronic low pack pain as a symptom of women wearing high heels.

Estimations indicate that the average American takes over 10,000 steps each day. That is more than 3.5 million steps each year. Compromising your feet, legs, pelvis and low back for glamour is a personal decision that should be reconsidered.

Quote of the week: *"You cannot shake hands with a closed fist."*—Golda Meir

High heels can cause knee problems

Question: My girlfriend wears 3-inch high heels and says it doesn't bother her. When I wear them my low back and knees get sore. Is there a relationship between low-back pain and knee problems and high heels?

Answer: Wearing any high-heeled shoes, both those with narrow heels or even with wider heels can potentially set a woman up for future arthritis in her knees and low back.

Wide high heels may appear to be easier on the feet and body more than narrow stiletto type heels, but they cause the same amount of abnormal torque (twisting) in the knees as well as increase lordorsis (forward curve) in the low back. The focus women put on their achy feet from their high heels tends to redirect their attention from the pains in their knees and back. It is the long-term routine cumulative wear and tear that causes damage to the knees and low back.

It is true, the higher the heel the more potential damage. Minimizing your heels to 2 inches or less will decrease chances of irritation. Any heel does cause torque and damage.

If you must be fashionable and chic then compensate for your style with regular stretching of the calves, hamstring, quadriceps and back muscles. Take your high heel shoes off whenever possible throughout the day, even while seated, to allow anatomical structures to relax. Should knee or low-back pain persist consider Chiropractic as a primary source to correct misaligned joints.

Quote of the week: *"Once you have learned to love, you will have learned to live."*—Unknown

Holistic health care is choice care of 21st century

Question: What is holistic health and holistic health care?

Answer: Holistic health care refers to the treatment of the whole body rather than just the symptoms of one condition. It refers to understanding that all functions and structures of the body work together. It refers to the fact that we are spiritual/physical/chemical and psychological—all in one—and each interacts with the other.

Holistic health care generally involves the use of alternative health measures such as Chiropractic, massage therapy, acupuncture, acupressure, homeopathy and others. Although holistic health care has been practiced for centuries, it has recently become an alternative to expensive and increasingly bureaucratic health-care systems.

Holistic health care uses a nurturing and empowering approach and makes the patient a partner in the healing process. Holistic health care takes a broad view of illness and disease by identifying multiple causes for the condition. It concentrates on healing the whole body as opposed to healing a particular disease. It attempts to perform non-invasive treatments that don't dictate the body's functions but rather supports them.

Holistic health care methods have become a viable alternative to depending on the drugs with their side effects and propensity for addiction. The fundamental basis of holistic health care is that your body knows best how to be well and just needs proper support.

Holistic health care has become the health care of the 21st century. It combines the best of modern diagnosis with the ancient remedies. These remedies include spinal adjustments, different types of "touch" therapy, nutritional supplements, herbal remedies, natural diets, exercise, mediation and breathing exercises, yoga and more. It addresses problems within the family and emphasizes prevention, wellness, maintenance and longevity. The patient is not just a passive recipient of health care but an active participant in a team effort.

Quote of the week: *"Do not ask people to do what you are not willing to do yourself."*—Phillip C. McGraw

How we stand has a direct effect on our spines

Question: I am a teenager and my mother is always telling me to stand up straight. Does how I stand really effect my spine?

Answer: Your mom is absolutely correct. In fact until you are emancipated your mom is always correct. She may want you to stand up straight because you look healthier and more mature. There are even more important reasons she doesn't even probably understand. Deviant postural habits such as sticking your one hip out with the hand and elbow sticking out to the side is a classic teenage girl stance. When you put yourself in any repetitive, consistent posture your brain and nervous system store a memory to that posture. Unfortunately, poor posture can register adaptive changes to the spine that irritate functions in the body and can design permanent growth changes.

Teenage women go through rapid growth spurts that will alter symmetry and balance in the spine, with poor posture, as it grows. As the twig grows, so follows the tree. A bent twig leads to a bent tree in nature. Scoliosis, a lateral bending or deviation in the spinal nerves is one result of the repetitive poor posture behaviors.

Standing, sitting, and walking with proper posture in mind are extremely helpful in minimizing postural distortions. Exercise, diet and regular spinal maintenance with Chiropractic care are the best tools to sustain the maximal potential of any teenager's healthy growth and posture.

My advice is listen to your mom, stand up straight, eat your vegetables and see your Chiropractor regularly.

Quote of the week: *"One love, one heart...let's get together...it will be all right."*—Bob Marley

How you carry pocketbook can create neck and/or back pain

Question: I carry a pocketbook over my shoulder for hours at a time and have neck and back irritation daily. Is there a more correct position and what are my alternatives?

Answer: A year ago I wrote a column about men wearing huge wallets in their back pockets and how the repetitive pressure on the buttock muscles and sciatic nerve can cause back and leg pain. You may recall the episode of "Seinfeld" where George has a monstrous wallet in his back pocket. A heavy pocketbook over the shoulder repetitively for any extended period of time has the same effect as a George-size wallet in the back pocket. Generally, your pocketbook strap, which in most cases are narrow, lye on the outer edge of your trapezious muscle as it inserts into the shoulder. Consistent pressure on this area pulls on the tendons, which attach your skull to your neck and shoulder. The muscles respond to steady pressure by contracting. The continual tightening of these muscles can create mild to even severe inflammatory responses as well as spasms, which may lead to headaches.

The alternatives to wearing a pocketbook are to wear a backpack or backpack style pocketbook. I was recently in Europe and it is very stylish for both men and women to wear these. Wearing a waist pouch is another less irritable means of carrying your necessary personal items. It is a good idea to periodically clean out heavy items from your pocketbook to lighten the load. Most women seem to believe they are about to be called for the next appearance of "Let's Make A Deal" and carry everything possible including a left-handed monkey wrench. The key is to have symmetry in the distribution of the weight you place upon your spine.

Any continued discomfort after making the appropriate adjustments may indicate a developing unhealthy condition, which should be checked by a Chiropractor.

Quote of the week: *"Nobody holds a good opinion of a man who has a low opinion of himself."*—Anthony Trollope

Hypochondriacs can be helped with group therapy

Question: My aunt always has something wrong with her. If it isn't her back, its headaches, stomach pain and many other symptoms. This is going on for over 15 years and I am convinced she is a hypochondriac. What can be done to help her?

Answer: Billions of dollars are spent by hypochondriacs on unnecessary diagnostic testing and doctor's visits yearly. According to Harvard Medical School research, hypochondriacs run up medical cost 15 percent.

Many physicians feel these type patients need psychological help. A study by the American Psychosomatic Society indicated that group therapy reduced medical costs by over $1,000 for those who participated in group therapy versus those that did not.

Clinically, we predominately see a direct link between patients emotional experiences and physical sensations. Obviously, not all patients are hypochondriacs; in fact my belief is none are. Some people just need to find the correct treatment medium to help conquer their problems.

Long-term physical stress can lead to emotional distress and long term psychological stress can lead to physical ailments.

There are those patients that refuse to let go of their fears, pains, and ailments. Many patients are their own worse enemy. I believe they must heal from within and spending enormous amounts of money on multitude of doctors is an expression of their inability to confront reality. Unfortunately, many of these patients end up on antidepressants. The drugs may help calm these patients and allow them to exist in society, but to be well they will have to combat themselves and let go.

Quote of the week: *"Victim of this, victim of that, your daddy's to thin and mommas' too fat. Get over it!"*—Eagles

Infant care—safe and smart

Question: My neighbor recently had a baby and she stopped at her Chiropractor's office on the way home from the hospital, even before seeing her relatives. She told me she had done this with her other two children and it made her feel secure that the newborn was getting off to a good start. Why would she be so emphatic about getting her newborn checked immediately by her Chiropractor?

Answer: Chiropractors check for subluxations which are tiny misalignments of the spine, cranium and pelvis which cause upset to the functioning of the baby's nerve system. These subluxations are by their very nature harmful and no other health professional is trained to detect them. Subluxations in the young do not result in pain. They can go completely unnoticed by the parent or they may express themselves subtly (as in a decreased immune response or decreased alertness) or they may express themselves overtly (as in the case of colic or ear problems).

Subluxations detected and corrected early will benefit not only the function (physiology) of the child but also the actual growth of the tissues and organs. The body remodels itself to stressors placed on it. As the newborn grows he or she will grow around or adapt to these early stresses. Some subluxations, if not corrected in the first year of life can never be fully corrected. At birth, there are supporting membranes within the cranium. These can be distorted by abnormal molding of the cranium caused either by unbalanced forces on the cranium before birth or by forces introduced during the birthing process. The reality is that these membranes grow into solid bone about the time of the baby's first birthday. If the corrections are not made in the first year, it will be impossible to fully correct the problem later.

All subluxations should be detected and corrected as soon as possible because if they are not, permanent damage to the joints themselves will occur.

Even if your baby had a very uneventful birth and looks and acts in a perfectly healthy manner, you should get your child checked by a Chiropractor for the previously mentioned reasons and these; babies have very heavy heads relative to the strength of their neck muscles and this predisposes them to neck subluxations. All babies statistically have a 50-percent chance of receiving a macro-trauma in their first year. Many times these accidents occur without your knowledge while your child is being watched by a baby sitter or relative. Babies also receive micro-trauma which is the cumulative effect of dozens of small jars and upsets that occur in learning to crawl, to sit, to stand, etc. Finally, the birth process itself is always a stress on the child's structure and therefore the main reason your neighbor was so bright and responsible to have her newborn's spine checked immediately after birth.

Quote of the week: *"One good wish changes nothing. One good decision changes everything."*—Anonymous

Innate intelligence and Chiropractic

Question: My question is one of a philosophical nature. After speaking with a friend in the Chiropractic college, the topic of innate intelligence came up. What is innate intelligence, and how does it relate to Chiropractic?

Answer: Innate intelligence has many synonyms, but they all mean the same. "Innate," the shortened term we use in Chiropractic, is the life force carried by the nervous system from above, down, and inside out. It flows through our bodies telling us how to grow, heal, live, and die.

Innate exists in every cell of our bodies and has inherent qualities that we cannot control. We can alter, irritate, enhance, or be in tune with our innate, but it will always exist.

If it sounds like a spiritual belief, in a way it is. Some people call the innate intelligence of the body God, life force, life blood, common energy, etc. One thing these terms have in agreement is that something does exist in our bodies that has intelligence, heals wounds, makes our hearts beat, converts food into fuel, and directs every other non-conscious functional effort.

When you cut yourself, do you have to think about the numerous reactions that are necessary to create a clot, draw the wound together, and then leave new, healthy skin? No. What if you are missing one factor in the intelligence to make a scab, as does a hemophiliac? You could bleed to death. Nurturing your innate and keeping the channels open so that it exists without interruption should be monitored for life.

Chiropractors remove barriers to the full expression of your innate intelligence. They do this by removing aberrant, irritated signals in the nervous system.

The nervous system is the physical conduit for transportation of the innate intelligence. Restoration of channels for the nervous system allows the innate to flow freely, creating greater expression of an individual's human potential.

Quote of the week: *"It is an endless and frivolous pursuit to act by any other rule than the one of satisfying our own minds in what we do."*—Richard Steele

Insurance coding complicated procedure

Question: I am confused about my insurance forms when I get my explanation of benefits (EOB) describing the payment for charges for my prior visits to my Chiropractor. Can you describe what the different codes and charges mean?

Answer: The insurance coding system for health care has become a science that requires a master's degree to decipher. It appears you need a medical degree with an accounting minor and specialty in health-care coding to understand the complicated and ever-changing practices of the health-care insurance industry. It is difficult for your doctor and his or her staff to make sense of the coding and reimbursement protocols, let alone you—the insured party—with a lay person's basic education.

My staff must take periodic update seminars and follow up on changes in the industry to maintain proper coding and procedures. Without exact documentation, precise coding and appropriate charges, the insurance carriers will deny or reduce a payment for a procedure code or a diagnosis code. Many times these denials will appear on the EOB mailed to you, the patient, prior to your physician seeing them. If you discard these EOBs without your physician's staff reviewing them it can delay proper payment for weeks to even months.

We cannot expect a patient to understand these denial codes and cryptic messages if we can't ourselves. Please keep them attached to your payment, copy them and bring them in for the physician's insurance staff to review and research.

The rising cost of health care is predominately due to the bureaucracy of tier review and mistake-ridden activities on the part of the carriers and physicians offices. There is an exceptional room for error due to data re-coding to computer transfer and multiple person handling.

Another challenge to the coding enigma is the doctor's accuracy of denoting correct codes for the procedures. The entire process will falter if the carrier doesn't recognize or reimburse for the procedure codes. Any early error becomes a cascade of denials and confusion.

The answer for you, the patient, when it comes to reviewing your EOBs is to:

1. have confidence in your physician and staff to be ethical and accurate and

2. to learn as much as possible about your personal health-care policy to be able to question your carrier with specific questions.

Quote of the week: *"Accept the challenges so that you may feel the exhilaration of victory."*—General George S. Patton

Jet lag helped by Chiropractic care

Question: I am traveling over Easter break and dread the jet lag after the long trip. What tips could you give me, and can Chiropractic help?

Answer: Jet lag is a very common symptom of travel for all people in all societies. The stress of travel is greater than ever before. You can't just go to the airport, get on a plane and fly to your destination. It takes almost as many hours of preparation and waiting as it does to drive in many cases. Preparation is essential for long flights to avoid jet lag.

Always try to get enough rest the night before your trip. Don't leave last second hurrying that can create stress and anxiety. Get to the airport very early. Drink plenty of water and have water available throughout your trip. Dehydration plays a large role in the effects of potential jet lag. Get up and walk around the cabin if it is safe. Stretch as often as possible. Support your back and neck so that you don't fall asleep in an unusual and uncomfortable position.

Chiropractic adjustments prior to and after arriving to your destination have proven to be very beneficial in minimizing jet lag. The results of a study in the *Journal of Manipulative and Physiological Therapeutics* indicated a positive effect that Chiropractic and had on athletes. From the perspective of mood, the Chiropractic-adjusted athletes had lower tension, anger, fatigue, and confusion than the sham-adjusted or control-group of athletes. In addition, the amount of vigor (energy) of the Chiropractic adjusted-athletes was higher than the sham-adjusted or control-group participants.

Quote of the week: *"People never improve unless they look to some standard or example higher and better than themselves."*—Tyron Edwards

Laughter heals

Question: My sister laughs at everything all the time and she says that is why she never gets sick. Is it true that laughing can keep you healthy?

Answer: Laughter is an essential part of health. Laughing keeps you healthy and diminishes illness by producing immunoglobulins (natural germ fighters). Laughter also allows the release of endorphins, our natural painkillers. Lung congestion conditions, such as asthma and bronchitis, respond well to laughing because it breaks up mucous and filtrates the exchanges of bad air and good air. Increased oxygen to the brain and body help clarity of thinking and cleanse the body of toxins.

The most obvious result of a good laugh is stress reduction. It is hard to be upset at the same time you are laughing. Children don't seem to carry stress loads as high as adults. This could be because the average child laughs sixty times a day while the average adult only laughs five times a day.

Laughter and its effects are being studied at institutions all over the planet. Even Harvard University has a laugh study center.

Your sister may seem silly but she is also very smart. If you are not laughing at her, better to laugh with her. In this case the last laugh is best.

Quote of the week: *"Flexible people never get bent out of shape."*—Anonymous

Love heals

Question: It is Valentine's Day this week and I have a question. I have seen it on TV and heard it from everyone, but is it just a cliché, or true, that "love heals"?

Answer: This sounds like a question for "Dear Abby", not me. I will do my best to reply in the vein of the physiological effects rather than psychological effects love has on us.

Physiologically when we feel better or loved we have a better immune system to fight disease and illness. Studies done on premature babies in incubators displayed marked recovery and response time for the newborns that were touched and had time spent with them as opposed to those not touched.

We also know those elevated feelings of love, joy and happiness are in direct proportion to balanced serotonin levels in the brain, which give us happiness levels. When serotonin levels are disturbed or are on a roller coaster of peaks and valleys, we can get emotionally depressed or general malaise.

We secrete endorphins when in love (our natural painkillers), therefore the cliché "lovers feel no pain". We secrete adrenaline when in love. Adrenaline is the natural glandular secretion for the production of energy. When in love we can't get enough out of life and our tone levels and expectations abound with excitement. We do not need any special elixirs, caffeine or energy supplements when in love. Love is Mother Nature's natural high.

Clinically, I observe patients in love and see an abundance of life in them. They walk with an aura of glow of bright light surrounding them. There is no substitute for love's effects on healing. The love of a pet or a child can cure and ailing soul.

In my personal and professional opinion, love heals everything and is the omnipotent force behind all living things.

I am not "Dear Abby," but I think she would agree that "love heals.". Don't ever stop giving or receiving love. Happy Valentines Day.

Quote of the week: *"Love is all you need."*—The Beatles

Lumbar-support belts stabilize the low back

Question: I recently injured my low aback and saw a Chiropractor help. He adjusted me and gave me therapies. My question is why did he give me a lumbar-support belt?

Answer: Every condition is unique and there area protocols for each type of condition. Along with your Chiropractor's clinical experience and professional knowledge, there is an innate sense of the best treatment in any situation. An acute low-back condition warrants immediate attention. R.I.C.E. is a good pneumonic to remember how to care for these conditions. R = Rest, I = Ice, C = Compression, and E = Elevation.

Lumbar-support belts fall in the category of compression. Initial injuries to the low back can potentially worsen with activity. My policy is to suggest the use of the binding action of the belts to minimize the activity of the muscles of the lumbar spine. I believe it is important to protect the spine initially but to restore activity as soon as possible. In most acute low-back muscle-oriented conditions our patients are weaning the usage of the belt by the third or fourth day and are told only to use them when they know they will be taxing those muscles for activity. Should a patient continue to wear his or her belt beyond the initial acute phase of injury it is very easy for the low-back muscles to lose tone and become dependent on the support.

You may have noticed that many of the employees at the home-improvement type stores wear support belts. This is very prudent of them and anyone that is working in an environment that requires heavy lifting at sporadic moments. Taking the low back from a relaxed state to a contracted state quickly, without preparation can create injury to the tissues. In these cases, wearing a low-back support can be preventative in nature.

Quote of the week: *"Experience is the name so many people give to their mistakes."*—Oscar Wilde

Many "myths" about low-back pain

Question: Is it true that once you get low-back problems you always have them? Is it also true that when you have a low-back history when you are younger, you can't walk very long periods when you get old?

Answer: The questions you are asking are commonly asked and part of a barrage of "myths" surrounding the generalized condition of low-back pain. When any type of physician is studying for his/her particular specialty there is a small percentage of students that develop a condition called "medical student syndrome," which is developing the condition you are studying. An example of this would be studying diabetes and then feeling numbness in your extremities even though there is no cause for the condition other than that the mind was convinced it had the condition. I bring this to light because I believe there is a similar condition with patients when they read or hear information, gossip, or stories about other patients with similar conditions and then believe or create the same condition for themselves.

Low-back pain is so unique to each individual that I suggest that no two people have the same condition. The definition of sciatica from *Dorland's Medical Dictionary* states, "A syndrome characterized by pain radiating from the back into the buttock and into the lower extremity or pain anywhere along the course of the sciatic nerve."

This common diagnosis is so vague that it can be misconstrued to mean almost any possible condition in the lower back or lower extremities. When patients claim they have the same low-back pain as their friend or neighbor, or low-back pain is in their family, I am very skeptical to agree. The "myth" that once you have low back, you will have it forever, is a premature illusion. You can definitely choose to have it forever or you can choose to correct it. Yes, there are a small percentage of patients that have unresolving low-back pain for years or their entire life, even after doing everything possible to relieve it. Most of our Chiropractic patients get low-back pain relief and more importantly low-back pain resolution and correction. Low-back pain that occurs in your youth has a greater chance of being corrected than long-established patterned low-back pain conditions. The earlier the cause of your pain is detected and corrected, the less likely you will have problems in the future or have difficulty with mobility.

My advice is to not wait for low-back pain and have your spine checked by a Chiropractor as part of your regular preventative maintenance. The integrity of your nervous system is essential to the vitality of your life. I am sure you get your teeth checked regularly, so it makes sense to get your spine checked regularly.

Quote of the week: *"An ounce of prevention is worth a pound of cure."*—Someone's Grandma

Massage and Chiropractic enter mainstream

Question: It seems there is a Chiropractor or massage therapist on every main street in the country. Why have these alternative health care providers become so popular?

Answer: A recent study published in the *Annals of Internal Medicine*, defined the role of complementary and alternative medical (CAM) therapies. The CAM therapies include massage and Chiropractic as the two must widely sought treatments.

The most revealing statistic was the effectiveness of alternative forms of care on the 10 most commonly reported ailments. Alternative care providers came out on top more often. CAM therapy was considered better for back conditions, arthritis, headaches, and neck conditions. Conventional medical care was considered superior for only hypertension.

The study, which questioned a sample group of 2,055 people, identified trends and consumer perceptions of health care. The bottom line reasons you see Chiropractors and massage therapists on every street corner is they make a substantial improvement for their patient's overall health and well being.

The summary of the study determined that consumers are increasingly using alternative care to address current ailments and improve overall health. It also stated consumers are spending their own money for Chiropractic and other forms of alternative care and are becoming more responsible for choosing which care is most appropriate for them. The trend is taking place in all parts of our society, is growing, and younger people will be driving this trend well into the future.

Medical doctors are no longer the dictators of health; they are just another team member.

Quote of the week: *"Hold yourself responsible for a higher standard than anybody else expects of you. Never excuse yourself."*—Henry Wood Beecher

Medical and Chiropractic philosophies differ drastically

Question: I recently had appointments with my medical doctor and Chiropractor on the same day. Their philosophies on health seemed almost totally opposite. What is the difference between "medical" and "Chiropractic" philosophies?

Answer: Let's look at the bottom line definition to answer your question immediately. "Medicine" is the study of disease and what causes a man to die while "Chiropractic" is the study of health and what causes a man to live.

Another definition or label for the medical model is Mechanistic (Rationalism) vs. the Chiropractic model Vitalism (Empiricism). Mechanists (rationalists) believe the body can be figured out using chemical, mathematical, or other disciplines. Mechanists like mechanisms and will often deny or criticize phenomena that conflict with (or cannot be explained by) "known" mechanism.

Vitalists (empiricists) admit that our knowledge is limited and we should be open to possibility of "surprises". That is why a vitalist healing art is a discovered one (example: Chiropractic, chelation therapy, etc.) while a mechanistic art is based on a theory (example: An aspirin a day and vaccination).

Modern medicine has become disconnected from the patient. The focus on diagnosis and understanding has evolved as primary concerns over usefulness to patient healing and cure. Modern Chiropractic maintains it's original premises which focus on the body's own innate intelligence and ability to heal itself respecting the fact that we are changing and adapting every second of every day. The principals of vitalism acknowledge that we are physically, mentally, and chemically in constant flux and any one area out of balance can alter the being as a whole.

It is time to accept that every individual is just that, an individual. We cannot treat human beings like cookbooks. Our health functions differ in various environments.

Every healing philosophy has its place and each exists to put checks and balances on the other. We all need each other and if we work together the benefactor will be you, the patient.

Quote of the week: *"Disease is the lack of coordination between innate, the source of power, and its expression."*—D. D. Palmer (founder of Chiropractic)

Medicare covers Chiropractic

Question: I am living in an adult retirement community and we have been discussing as to whether Chiropractic treatment is or is not covered by Medicare. Could you clarify if Medicare covers Chiropractic?

Answer: Medicare absolutely covers Chiropractic care. The misunderstanding may be that some Chiropractors may participate with Medicare and some may not. It is the option of the doctor to choose whether or not they will accept the Medicare guidelines in their practice. Presently, Medicare covers 12 visits to the Chiropractor a year. If your Chiropractor feels you are required to have more, he or she can appeal to Medicare with the special circumstances and examination findings that verify the need for additional care beyond the allotted 12 visits. X-rays for Medicare patients may be taken at the Chiropractor's office, but may not be covered.

Many of our Medicare patients have a second insurance, which covers the difference of what Medicare does not cover. Once you receive an explanation of benefits, outlining what was covered and what treatment was denied you can submit the difference to your secondary insurance company and they should pay it in most cases.

Even with modern technology such as electronic billing, it may take from 4 to 6 weeks before Medicare sends its' first explanation of benefits and/or a check to your doctor.

Our Medicare patients have been very successful with Chiropractic care. It is the best alternative treatment for the elderly. It restores motion back to the joints and increases mobility. Many elderly people don't realize they have this great opportunity for Chiropractic service. I hope you are better informed so you can tell your friends.

Quote of the week: *"We are what we repeatedly do. Excellence, then, is not an act but a habit."*—Anonymous

Mid-back pain is a serious condition

Question: Most of my friends complain about their low-back pain or neck pain. My pain is in the mid-back and never seems to go away. Is mid-back pain as severe a problem as neck or low-back pain?

Answer: Any spinal pain is a serious concern. There is no scale to measure what part of the spine or what degree of pain is a more serious condition. Every individual has a specific response to a specific trauma to the spine. Some people are inherently more resilient and more adaptive.

Thoracic or mid-back spinal conditions create an added challenge because of the attachment of ribs to the vertebra. The thoracic region is designed to protect the body's vital organs. The combination of spine, ribs, and sternum create a strong and stable enclosure, the combination also prohibits much movement in the thoracic spine.

Because movement in the thoracic spine is limited, it is less susceptible to degenerative disease, herniated discs, instability, or other problems more common to the lumbar or cervical spine. Common causes of mid-back pain include poor posture, muscle irritation, or exposure to repetitive stress. A common cause is leaning forward at the computer for extended times.

Thoracic vertebra have a tendency to fixate due to their minimal motion. Attempting movement against the locked or fixated joints can continually re-aggravate the condition.

Specific Chiropractic adjustments can release these fixations gently and painlessly in most cases. Additional or corresponding treatment with physiotherapies such as ice, ultrasound, electric stimulation, and massage are also helpful.

Quote of the week: *"The same heart beats in every human breast."*—Matthew Arnold

Mood swings helped by Chiropractic care

Question: Can Chiropractic help with my symptoms? I suffer with every menstrual cycle. I get bloated, cramping, severe mood swings and crankiness as well as low-back pain.

Answer: Chiropractic has shown to be effective in minimizing if not eliminating many of your types of symptoms related to menstruation. Many women suffer with similar symptoms and have been under the misunderstanding that these symptoms are normal. These symptoms are not normal.

Many pregnant patients with a variety of these symptoms also seek Chiropractic care. Pregnancy and menstruation cycle are two of the most important health matters for women. Pregnancy and its recovery, pain during the menstrual period (dysmennorrhea), premenstrual syndrome (PMS), and chronic pelvic pain are four of the most distressing conditions that are unique to the female body that Chiropractic can help you with.

Chiropractors educate women in diet, nutrition, weight loss, methods for maintaining wellness and general fitness. More importantly, Chiropractors use gentle procedures and have a caring interaction with the concerns a woman has during these periods of their life.

Adjustments to specific misaligned vertebra (subluxation) will allow for proper nerve supply to improperly functioning tissue. A common area of subluxation for women with menstrual problems is the lumbar-sacral and sacroiliac regions. These areas send direct nerve supply to the reproductive tissue and effect the glands, which effect normal balance.

The correction of subluxations is the specialty of Chiropractors. A thorough history, complete examination and diagnostic testing which may include X-rays can detect the cause of your problem.

My advice is not to hesitate in getting an evaluation since so much success has been revealed for your condition.

Quote of the week: *"Great minds must be ready not only to take opportunities but to make them."*—Colton

Movement for infants is vital

Question: I have an infant whom spends a lot of time in a car seat and carrier as we do our daily activities. Is it harmful for her to spend so much time seated at her age?

Answer: Humans are meant to move and play. Babies, in fact spend nearly half of their waking time—40 percent—doing things like kicking, bouncing, and waving their arms. While it may appear all the activity a baby performs is just for the sake of "just moving" or "just playing," every action extends a child's development in some way.

Infant's movement capabilities are extremely limited when compared with even those of a toddler, but movement experiences may be more important for infants than for children of any other age group. Thanks to new insights in brain research, we now know that early movement experiences are considered essential to the neural stimulation needed for healthy development.

An infant's brain is full of brain cells (neurons) at birth. In fact a 1-pound fetus has 100 billion of them! Over time each of these brain cells can form as many as 15,000 connections (synapses) with other brain cells. It is during the first 3 years of life that most of these connections are made. Research indicates that physical activity and play during early childhood have a vital role in the sensory and physiological stimulation that results in more synapses. Physical movement, from the earliest infancy and throughout our lives, plays an important role in the creation of nerve cell networks, which are actually the essence of learning.

Gross and fine-motor skills are learned through repetition as well. Repetitive movement lays down patterns in the brain.

Unfortunately our society trends are indicating infants are spending upward of 60 waking-hours a week in restraints such as high chairs, carriers, car seats and the like. Being confined affects a baby's personality.

Baby's need to be held also. Extended restraint may also have serious consequences for the child's motor and cognitive development.

If your infant has any unusual behavior or signs of abhorrent movements they should be checked by a Chiropractor who understands how neurological interruption can interfere with function.

Quote of the week: *"Babies are such a nice way to start people"*—Don Herold

Musicians must be careful of posture

Question: My son has been taking guitar lessons for a year now and it seems his back hurts the more he plays. Do you have any suggestions for him to prevent his discomfort?

Answer: Historically many musicians, especially classical string instrument performers, have back conditions. Many instruments do not lend themselves to a posturally balanced spine. Bending forward, rotated with your head slightly flexed is a common position for guitar players. In this position weight bearing is generated to the upper back. Although these muscles are strong, they can get overdeveloped and create asymmetries in the posture which re-distribute pressure to sensitive soft tissue and nerves surrounding the spine. The result is pain and discomfort. Professional musicians that perform or practice for hours a day should have a strong commitment to maintaining appropriate posture and take active measures on a daily basis to counter effect the habitual positions that their instrument burdens them with. This same advice holds true for a beginning musician. Developing good warm up and stretching regiments can definitely minimize back irritation.

Many amateur and professional musicians choose Chiropractic care as their means of balance and correction of irritation secondary to playing. A Chiropractor can identify the abhorrent position and give ideas on how to make adjustments.

A study in the magazine *Clinical Chiropractic* questioned over 107 musicians and discovered that there is a high rate of injury to professional classical musicians and teachers. A majority of those interviewed felt that their injuries were disruptive to practice and potentially threatening to their careers.

The incorporation of postural and ergonomic considerations into musical education along with Chiropractic treatment programs can be of benefit to both teachers and students.

Quote of the week: *"Faith is the antiseptic of the soul."*—Walt Whitman

Nation is getting sicker

Question: It seems to me more people are sicker than ever. Every winter more of my friends and family around the country are worse off health wise than the year before. Why is everyone getting so ill, even with all our advanced technologies?

Answer: You are not imagining that the nation is getting sicker. We are getting very ill as a nation in general. A recent public survey conducted by the United Health Foundation, measuring health indicators, found a 3-percent decline in "relative healthiness of the American population." It is the largest drop in the nation's overall health in the 12-year history of the report. The report blames the rise on increases in cigarette smoking, a drop in high school graduations, and an increase in premature deaths.

Observing friends, neighbors, and family you can see health changes worsen due to poor personal habits and hygiene. Over eating and obesity are abundant especially in school children. Decreased exercise and minimal gym requirements in schools have allowed children to avoid even minimal activity. Combine over eating with under activity and you have an equation that equals health disaster. As bad as this poor-health model is for children it is even more devastating for adults. Increased television and computer time diminish activity time. Excessive sitting hampers the spinal functions and interferes with healthy nerve function.

The study indicated that the states with the lowest health scores included: Louisiana, Mississippi, South Carolina, West Virginia, and Florida. Those with the highest: Minnesota, New Hampshire, Utah, Connecticut, and Massachusetts.

Americans need to get off their butts and start being responsible for their own health. Stop being dependent on drugs, vitamins, doctors, health gurus and gadgets. Health comes from above down inside out. So, tell your friends and family to go out for a walk and don't forget to smell the roses.

Quote of the week: *"You bring the beauty to the rose."*—B.J. Palmer

Natural sunlight is healthier than artificial

Question: I have heard that artificial light is really bad for your skin and health. Is natural sunlight better for you heath than tanning salon lights?

Answer: Our skin is made to enjoy the sun. When you body is not healthy enough to benefit from the sun, is when we have problems. Many people that have skin and health problems from the sun are those that abuse themselves through over-exposure. Too much sun without coverage such as just wearing a bathing suit for hours at a time or even days at a time can cause damage to the skin. Spending a lot of time outdoors in the sun is normal and healthy especially if it is during an activity. A weak immune system either from a poor diet or stress, will make you vulnerable to sun damage and disease.

Avoiding sunburn at any age, but especially early in life, is a key to preventing skin cancers later in life, especially melanoma, perhaps the most serious form of skin cancer. Unfortunately studies show that significant numbers of children still experience sunburn.

While the sun gives us nutrients and other benefits, it can also use up nutrients. Consider that sunlight helps control stress as well as sunlight on the body and its stimulation through the eyes actually influences the adrenal stress hormones in a positive way. In winter, a sunny day can be very therapeutic, and prevent and treat the common problem of Seasonal Affective Disorder (SAD). Throughout the year, the sun hitting your skin produces natural vitamin D. A healthy diet high in vegetable and some fruit is also high in natural antioxidants and other photo nutrients. These nutrients are vital in normal environmental adaptation, especially the sun's rays.

The natural darkness or pigment of you skin determines exposure sensitivity to the sun. Pale or light colored skin pigment is much more susceptible to skin damage than dark pigmented skin tones.

Some drugs can significantly increase your sensitivity to the sun. These include NSAIDS, certain antibiotics and antifungals, diuretics, various psychiatric drugs, and many others. Check with you pharmacist for specific information.

As far as tanning salons being less harmful to your skin, consider this. If your body is not capable of adapting the ultra-violet (UV) light, even mild exposure from salon devices can do considerable harm, including increased cancer risk and sunburn. Studies have shown the hazards of exposure by combining commercial tanning salon devices with even mild exposure to natural sunlight. If you use a tanning salon, make sure you provide you skin with the nutrients necessary to properly adapt to the artificial light like it would to natural exposure.

When using sunscreen use the most natural available for those times you have to be in the sun for long period and apply to most vulnerable areas.

Quote of the week: *"You make a living by what you do; you make a life by what you give."*—Winston Churchill

Neck and head injuries are severe

Question: I am a surfer and have a question. Why are people always so concerned about neck injuries like when you hit your head into the sand after coming off a wave?

Answer: Neck injuries as well as head injuries are extremely dangerous. The average head weighs approximately 8 pounds. The entire weight of your head rests on a vertebra called the "Atlas" or first cervical vertebra. The name Atlas implies the entire weight of the world. This is true in that the head is balanced on this vertebra and if this atlas vertebra is shifted out of position by a trauma or even light injury, the nerves between the head and the atlas can be irritated.

The nerves between the head and neck are vital in that they're sending information to the entire region of your head and neck including eyes, ears, nose and throat.

More important than the pair of spinal nerves exiting the upper cervical area, is the fact that your brain stem extends beyond your skull down to the 1st and 2nd vertebrae. You have vital brain sensitive tissue under your first two mobile vertebrae. This means that an injury to your neck could tear, inure or inflame your brain. Once brain damage occurs in this area it is often irreparable.

These sensitive brain stem areas control motor functions to a majority of your extremities and other joints and soft tissues in your body. A splintered fracture of one of these first two vertebras causing the bone to tear spinal nerves or brain tissue is next to impossible to repair because of the high concentration of neurons (nerve cells) in that area. There are literally millions of nerve impulses traveling to and from the nervous system every second of every day. An example of how fragile and intricate this area can be seen with the unfortunate horseback riding injury actor Christopher Reeves received. Reconnecting the severed nerve supply in this area is much more complicated than reattaching a severed arm. The concentration of nerve tissue diminishes as you move away from the spine.

What this all means to you as a surfer dude, is that yes, a head or neck injury is dangerous and you should protect your neck and head at all times.

Should you receive a severe neck or head injury it should be treated as an emergency situation. When severe injuries have been ruled out, correction of any misaligned vertebra in your spine should be analyzed by a trained Chiropractor.

Quote of the Week: *"The most terrifying thing is to accept yourself completely."*—Carl Sung

Nerve conduction testing is beneficial diagnostic tool

Question: My Chiropractor told me it was necessary to get nerve conduction velocity (NCV) and electromyography (EMG) testing done to determine how severe my nerve damage was. What are these tests and what do they tell you?

Answer: An NCV is a test for neuropathies, which are peripheral nerve damage. An NCV measures the speed and strength of nerve conduction once the nerve is stimulated. Theses tests along with other clinical criteria can assist in diagnosing the source of a patient's nerve interference and the degree to which it is damaged. These types of tests are used to differentially diagnose neuropathy conditions such as carpal tunnel, tarsal tunnel and many other radiculopathies.

An EMG is used to help detect loss of neurons enervating to a muscle. An EMG is also used to isolate radiuculopathies and is helpful in differentially diagnosing nerve root compression, herniated discs and peripheral nerve damage.

Needle EMG's may be slightly uncomfortable to the patient when performed because an impulse must pass into the muscle. NCV's are usually painless. Both tests take approximately 45 minutes to perform per upper or lower area tested. Results can be interpreted immediately. Remember, no test is the answer to a diagnostic question when used alone. A patient's history of injury and treatment along with corresponding testing makes for the most accurate diagnosis.

Quote of the week: *"True love doesn't have a happy ending: true love has no ending."*—Ed Mckenzie

Nerve injuries cause immune system suppression

Question: Ever since my accident to my neck, my nervous system has been malfunctioning. I know this because my ability to fight colds is terrible now. What is the relationship between my nervous system and immune system?

Answer: Science has continually been pouring out research supporting the fact that the nervous system is directly related to the proper function of the immune system. This is of particular importance when you understand that your immune system dictates your success or failure in adapting to your environment and also explains why some people seem to come down with every "little bug" while those around them are rarely ill.

Research at the University of Miami reported evidence suggesting that depression of immune function occurs early after spinal cord injury and is maintained there after. The most likely cause of immune abnormality was the decentralization of the nervous system. Additional factors causing immune depression include, over exposure to drugs or alcohol, medications, and fat rich diets.

Dr. Pero, another spinal researcher, conducted studies on the relationship of spinal nerve pressure and immune function. His finding concluded that those with the best spinal care habits had superior immune system function when compared to other groups not engaged in spinal care activities.

The Chiropractic profession is the largest group of healthcare professionals concerned with spinal care. While Chiropractic is great for aches and pains, it is now evident that it is equally as effective for helping to keep your nervous system and your immune system functioning at their highest levels, allowing you to express the greatest degree of health, naturally.

Quote of the week: *"Success doesn't come to you...you go to get it."*—Marua Collins

Nutrition and Chiropractic are good alternatives to hormone replacement

Question: I was stunned to read in the *New York Times* that hormone replacement was more dangerous than helpful. The article didn't give alternatives to the therapy. What could you suggest as an alternative to hormone-replacement therapy for women?

Answer: I am very aware of the article and news releases regarding the dangers of hormone replacement therapy. The study mentions that over 6 million women across the United States utilize hormone-replacement therapy. The in depth study discovered that drugs, a combination of estrogen and progestin caused small increases in breast cancer, heart attacks, and strokes and blood clots. Those risks outweighed the drugs' benefits, a small decrease in hip fractures and a decrease in colorectal cancer.

The study, supported by the National Institutes of Health, sent letters to many of the 16,000 women in the study, telling them to discontinue the drugs in light of the results.

A large concern of many women is what will be consequences of suddenly stopping to answer this question and your question regarding alternatives let us examine why these drugs are given in the first place. Until recently medical authorities were telling doctors to encourage almost every woman to start taking hormone-replacement drugs when she reached menopause, and to take them for years, even for life. Their purpose was to reduce the natural side effects that come with some women's menopause, including torrential night sweats, embarrassing hot flashes, moodiness, and depression. The most common reason that doctors encouraged the drug regime was to prevent osteoporosis, which is a progression of demineralization of bone tissue.

Considering the symptoms the drug regimes intended to correct, we have found that there can be coinciding or other causes of these side effects. Nutritionally, it has been demonstrated that supplementation of the appropriate amount of calcium-magnesium in the diet as well as Vitamin E has been successful in combating the menopausal symptoms. A proper diet, avoiding caffeinated beverages and high sugar concentrated products, support natural progression through menopause.

Chiropractically, we have a lot of success when neurological disturbed energy flow to the reproductive area is corrected through adjustments to the pelvis and lumbar spine.

You can't stop Mother Nature but you can assist her in naturally progression through what can be a difficult time for some women. If you have severe or persistent symptoms you should absolutely consult your own physician before replacing or stopping drug treatment.

Quote of the week: *"If there's a way to do it better...find it."*—Thomas Edison

Osteoporosis helped by Chiropractic

Question: I am 80-years-old and have been diagnosed with osteoporosis. Can I still be treated by a Chiropractor for my low-back and neck pain?

Answer: Osteoporosis can be treated by a Chiropractor as long as the degree of osteoporosis has been determined through diagnostic testing. Osteoporosis by definition is demineralization of bone. The density or thickness of bone is dependent upon the amount of minerals and vitamins stored within its cells. Osteoporosis is more common in postmenopausal women, chronic smokers, post traumatic conditions and patients with poor dietary habits. Osteoporosis is a slow and normal progression of aging. Most patients that have mild or moderate conditions will never know they have it and manage their lives asymptomatically. Severe or advanced osteoporosis may leave the body feeling weak, unstable and painful.

Chiropractors have to be careful treating patients with severe osteoporosis because the patient may have weak brittle bones. Aggressive or forceful adjusting is not recommended obviously in these cases. Gentle force techniques are not only advisable but tremendously helpful. Always let your doctor know if you have a history of osteoporosis. It can be detected with X-ray, magnetic-resonance imaging (MRI), computed tomography (CT) scan, and a bone-density scan.

Besides Chiropractic, nutritional supplementation of calcium, magnesium and multi-minerals are highly recommended. Increased water intake is imperative. You should always check with your personal physician before taking any supplement randomly. They can help you determine dosage and cater support to you as an individual.

Quote of the week: *"No matter how many times you have been wronged or hurt by others, all it takes is one act of kindness to make you believe in the goodness that exists in the world."*—Fredrick Wryer, Sr.

Overuse of painkillers can cause pain

Question: I have been taking painkiller medication for a chronic headache on and off for months now. The only time it seems I get pain relief is when I go off the medication. Is it possible the medication is causing the headaches and can Chiropractic help instead?

Answer: As a Chiropractor I will not tell you to take medication nor reduce medication for any condition. I can give you information regarding a study on chronic long-term analgesic intake for pain. A study released on May 11, 2004 in an issue of *Neurology* stated that daily or near daily use of analgesics is associated with chronic headaches, especially migraines, and to a lesser extent, with other chronic pain conditions, such as neck and back pain.

The International Headache Society defines "medication overuse headache" (MOH) as "headache appearing at least 15 days/month; regular intake of analgesics; and headache disappearing after withdrawal of substance." Some studies suggest that a startling 50-percent of cases of chronic headache are attributed to medication overuse.

I suggest you discuss your condition with your physician that prescribed your medication. There are over hundreds of causes of a headache and every individual expresses their condition uniquely. Taking the same medication or doing the same self-treatment a friend or peer did for their condition because it sounded like the same symptoms is very precarious.

Chiropractors are concerned with the cause of disease and will examine your spine and neurological function to determine if there is a relationship to your pain or headaches. Removal of nerve interference with specific gentle Chiropractic adjustments is extremely successful in correcting many of the causes of headaches. I highly suggest you consider a thorough consultation and examination with a Chiropractor to gain knowledge as to how you may be helped.

Quote of the week: *"There are two ways to live your life. One is as though nothing is a miracle. The other is as though everything is a miracle."*—Albert Einstein

Pain can be transferred to opposite ends of the spine

Question: Why would my Chiropractor look at my lower back after I told him that my pain was at the back of my skull?

Answer: The body, as well as the spine, is a living dynamic organism that is in constant adaptation to its environment. Every action, thought or movement has a reaction to that change. The body was designed to be perfect and maintain a homeostasis or balance. When patients present themselves to a Chiropractor it is the job of the Chiropractor to evaluate the entire person and not just the pain itself. The medical model of treating patients is more oriented to "cookbook conditions," meaning if a patient presents themselves with a specific symptom you give them a specific drug.

The Chiropractic and holistic approach focuses on the entire human being and approaches the symptom as a message to the body that something is wrong. It is not a bad thing but a protective mechanism of the body telling us that something is not in balance. In the case where the posterior of your head was sore and the Chiropractor looked at your lower spine has credence in this evaluation. Not only does the entire body have reaction to certain responses but also there is an equal and adaptive behaviors of the spine to each change. Doctors of Chiropractic understand that the spine adapts to upper-cervical and occipital movement by adapting the lower-lumbar and sacral segments of the spine. What this means is that whenever your head goes forward your buttock goes backward and visa versa. What is surprising about the nervous system and its response to long-term chronic irritation is that it minimizes the pain in small increments until we live with the discomfort and accept that it is normal. It is not until what appears to be a new symptom arises in another area that we take notice. Many times I have found that if the patients condition was not induced by trauma and the new symptoms just appeared suddenly the new symptoms are an adaptation for some other condition that has been masked for a long period of time. Acknowledging that opposite ends adapt to long-term conditions it is actually more common for the problem to stem from the opposite end of your spine than where the recent symptoms are.

Quote of the week: *"The unnatural—that too is natural."*—Goeth

Pain-killer medications have high risk for back-pain control

Question: I am very confused as to whether it is safe to take pain medication for my low-back pain. What are the risks and alternatives to taking these types of medications?

Answer: Recent studies revealed there is a one-in-50 chance that a male aged 65 to 74 will have a heart attack this year from taking either Celebrex, Vioxx, or Bextra and the percentage increases fivefold with high doses of Vioxx. These are the facts in a nutshell, based on all the publicity in the media. The problem is that even with the exposure of these high risks the U.S. Food and Drug Administration (FDA) hired a panel of experts that decided it was still safe to keep these pain-killer medications on the market. The 32-member committee voted February 18, 2005 that the benefits of Merck's Vioxx and Pfizer's Celebrex and Bextra outweighed the risk of cardiac damage. The *New York Times* reported on February 26, 2005 that the 10 panelists had financial ties to the two companies and a third maker of similar medicines. Without their votes, the findings would have been reversed for Vioxx and Bextra. The FDA obviously included a panel with conflicts in interest to satisfy their ambitions at the stake of integrity and safety to you the consumer. These types of actions are taken regularly in the drug industry, which represents the largest, wealthiest, and most influential lobbying body in our country.

It is your own personal responsibility to investigate and gain knowledge of every medication suggested to you and research its potential side effects. Utilize the Internet and call your physician before taking any pain-killer medication. Our government is taking a hands-off policy to monitoring medications and leaving all the liability to the individual drug companies as it appears.

Chiropractic can be an excellent alternative to the use of pain medication for back pain. Once appropriate adjustments of the spine are made and muscles are relaxed with therapies, pain reduction is significant in many pain-causing low-back conditions. Extreme or persistent pain may require medical intervention and your Chiropractor is trained to determine at what point a referral or emergency intervention is necessary.

Quote of the week: *"Oftentimes it is the thing we fear the most that we unconsciously bring about."*—Bessie J. Powell

Pain thresholds vary due to natural chemicals

Question: How can it be that my husband can withstand pain after injuries and during viruses while I suffer excessively with the same type of exposures?

Answer: We all have different pain thresholds. There are many different theories on why this occurs. Some researchers propose that we are born with different natural abilities to neutralize pain while other researchers feel we develop our abilities to combat pain through our life experiences and exposures.

A study by Dr. Jon-Kar Zubieta, et al., 2001, offers insight into the way the human body dampens pain, by producing and wielding natural opioids such as endorphins and enkephalins. The study demonstrated that the painful stimulus caused the notable opioid activity in regions of the brain associated with sensation and emotion. The experimental subjects demonstrated great individual variability in their response to pain, though all had pain stimulus of similar intensity. And the response correlated with activation of the opiod system (pain receptors in the brain)

Dr. Zubeta concluded, "This may help explain why some people are more sensitive, or less sensitive, than others when it comes to painful sensations. We show that people vary both in number of receptors that they have for these anti-brain chemicals, and in their ability to release the anti-pain chemicals themselves."

Both these factors apparently determine emotional and sensory aspects of a painful experience. These variations may explain why some people respond to pain medication and some don't. It may also explain why some people develop chronic pain conditions and others don't.

Quote of the week: *"Yesterday's endings are seeds for today's beginnings."*—Lewis Losoncy

Pets help heal their owners

Question: Is it true that animals are used to help heal people and does having a pet make you healthier?

Answer: All living species on our planet have a special niche and appropriate place in the big cosmic flow. Animals share this earth with us and their interaction is a vital part of life. Even at this very moment we are still learning about how important our animal friends can be in understanding human functions as well as how our environment changes.

Research on sea creatures such as sharks and dolphins is giving us a greater understanding of how sonar works and how communication systems are set up. Dolphin studies have been on-going for years in regards to their healing potential for humans.

At home we have discovered the tremendous healing capacity of pets. Pets can benefit our mental and our physical health. Reduction of stress is the greatest benefit. Studies have shown that pet owners have lover blood pressure and lower cholesterol levels. In general, this puts those who share their lives with animals at a reduced risk of heart disease.

A 10-month study that compared pet owners with non-pet owners found that the pet owners have fewer headaches, fewer bouts of indigestion, and less difficulty sleeping. The study ruled out increase in exercise but does bring to light another benefit of dog owners. One researcher who focused on this subject found that the average dog owner spends more than an hour a day outdoors with his or her animal. Fresh air and a brisk walk while relaxing your mind from all its stressful concerns is a tremendous mind and body enhancer.

Dogs and other pets act as built in motivators. Whether it is to wake you up each morning as a daily reminder to be fed or to be walked, pets keep us going and aide as perfect friends. An animal's healing non-judgmental love can add that special warmth to any household. Pets enrich our lives and give us a sense of optimism, safeguard us from depression and loneliness, as well as heal us psychologically and physically.

Quote of the week: *"Do not follow where the path may lead. Go instead where there is no path and leave a trail."*—Unknown

Poor eating habits damage health

Question: My mom says I am always sick because of my eating habits. I think what I eat is healthy. So, could she be right about my eating habits making me feel sick?

Answer: Moms are always right. Eating habits are even more important than what you eat. Bad eating habits include: eating on the run, eating too quickly without chewing your food, doing multiple tasks while trying to eat, eating too little or not at all, waiting until evening to eat a big meal, and many others.

A bad habit, I alert my patients about, is drinking too many fluids during meals. Excess fluid while eating dilutes your digestive enzymes not allowing your digestive tract to break down the food completely. Small sips are more advisable to create the breakdown of the food in the mouth and stomach.

Symptoms of poor eating habits include indigestion, flatulence (gas), aggravation of stomach and duodenal ulcers, aggravation of some hiatal hernias, diarrhea, and constipation. Additionally, poor eating habits also cause lost nutrients because the body either doesn't receive adequate nutrition or it does not have time to prepare the food for the maximum nutrient absorption.

If you only snack or completely skip a meal, you will probably notice later your body's reaction to your transgression. Symptoms resulting from meal skipping include the obvious stomach rumblings, headaches, weakness, light-headedness, and fatigue. Improper diet may also lead to the slowed healing of injuries.

A poor diet may not provide the vitamins and minerals needed for healing. Make eating a reverent experience. Savor each bite, relax, and enjoy the food. Allow each swallow to move completely into the stomach before taking another bite or drinking anything. Create a cycle of chewing and swallowing rather than continuous line of swallowing.

Quote of the week: *"He who has peace of mind disturbs neither himself nor another."*—Anonymous

Potential law suits mean more paperwork

Question: Last week I returned to see my Chiropractor after four years of no treatment. I was astounded at the amount of paperwork it took to fill out prior to my exam. Why is there so much paperwork needed these days?

Answer: The main reason your doctor and all doctors all over our country are requiring more data and records as well as signed notices, is that we live in a litigious society. Most paperwork is for prevention of lawsuits from the patients, insurance companies, malpractice and government business laws.

In the last 5 years, rigid standards and protocols have been put on hospitals, small practices and individual physicians. Public advocates, in their attempt to protect the public's interests, require disclosure of the intentions of the physician and any referrals he makes. Government insurance agencies such as Medicare and Medicaid change their policies on a regular basis and many of these changes require the doctor or facility to inform their patients by signing forms. The new Medicare Privacy Acts have now changed how health facilities conduct their business with the public. Compliance manuals have been required of all health-care facilities since September 2002.

This means even additional forms for the patient. I could not believe anyone, including the doctors' staff nor the patient, enjoy all this extra paperwork, but the bottom line is, it is required. If not performed, the doctor is legally bound by it and could be fined if not performing it appropriately. The doctor can now have his patients' records and files audited randomly by insurance companies and if they are not in compliance with accurate record keeping could have their payments rescinded.

The true paperwork that is time consuming but very important is a comprehensive health history. All healthcare practitioners should be responsible for requesting this history and reviewing it thoroughly with their patient prior to treatment. A thorough health history can be more revealing than the examination. It helps the patient identify where their condition may have originated.

If you feel the pain you have in your body is not as bad as the pain in filling out the doctors forms you are not alone. Until a better method arrives we must all comply, understanding this is for the protection and betterment of you the patient and your physician.

Quote of the week: *"When you come to a fork in the road, take it."*—Yogi Berra

Preparation prevents sports injuries

Question: Every basketball season my son pulls a hamstring in one of the first games. What can he do to prevent early season injuries?

Answer: Preparation and conditioning reduce injuries early in the athletic season and throughout the lifetime of a young or developed athlete.

Always prepare your cardiovascular system. Even young athletes need to have endurance and lung power. Always build your endurance on a steady gradient. You may want to start 2-to 3-months prior to your sporting season, unless you cross train year round. Walking, treadmill, biking, and swimming develop increased lung capacity.

Stretching all the musculoskeletal system (muscles, ligaments, and joints) increases full ranges of motion and elongates soft tissue. Early preparation prevents sprain/strain injuries when sudden extreme jolts or traumas occur.

Know your sport and know which muscles have more demand for utilization. For example tennis and basketball require a high degree of foot pivoting so stretch the ankles and knees by isolating the calf, hamstring, quadriceps and anterior leg muscles. Team coaches, trainers or Chiropractors are great places to start for information and guidance.

Most young athletes don't need to over tax their joints with excessive heavy weight lifting. Before the age of 18 most secondary growth centers are not fully established making joints prone to permanent injuries especially with repetitive heavy weight training.

Use common sense and don't utilize a joint or muscles if it gives you persistent pain or restriction. Consult a sports-injury specialist such as a Chiropractor.

Quote of the week: *"Everything we live through leaves some mark on us."*—Eugene Ionesco

Prepare prior to morning stretching

Question: Is morning stretching safe for my back as soon as I wake up?

Answer: Stretching for your spine and entire body is very important for a daily maintenance of your general health. The time of the morning you choose to do your stretching does make a difference. Any exercise or stretching immediately after waking up is discouraged due to the lack of circulation and metabolic preparedness. While you are sleeping your metabolism slows down, allowing all your organs and tissues to rest. Circulation slows down and blood in your muscles is fairly stagnant. Your brain and body work together to heal your tissues while you sleep. Enriched fluids filled with minerals and vitamins are sent to irritated areas as a healing mechanism of your innate intelligence. Areas of heat in the body attract these inflammatory elements and as a result engorge the irritated areas. The fluids will stay in these areas until you awake and start moving. The reason exercising immediately after waking is potentially harmful is that your muscles and joints are still full of theses fluids and they may feel stiff and uncomfortable causing you to over stretch tearing tissue. As you move the static fluid is dissipated out of the joints and tissues.

Taking a shower or waiting approximately a half hour is appropriate for most people. Teenagers and young children can usually jump out of bed and run around instantly because they have such quick metabolisms.

People that wake up in pain or take hours to have the stiff sensation leave their bodies may have a problem that needs attention. Rheumatoid arthritis gives these types of symptoms due to its fluid retention nature.

Daily spinal stretching is highly advised, only after allowing a period of adaptation. Should pain or stiffness persist you should consult your local Chiropractor.

Quote of the week: *"You never lose by loving. You always lose by holding back."*—Anonymous

Prevention is best policy to avoid injuries around the house

Question: I have injured my low back two times after falls at my home. What suggestions can you give to avoid slip and fall injuries?

Answer: Most slip and fall injuries occur on wet flooring, usually in the bathroom or kitchen. When your feet slide out from underneath you your most common landing zones are your buttocks or head. Grabbing for the floor with your hands is common and this may result in a wrist or elbow injury. Anti-slip surfaces do help, but once moisture is on a flat surface, especially without prior knowledge, danger lurks. Prevention in these situations of wet flooring would be to make sure you don't have any leaks or wet surfaces on a regular basis. When you notice a problem area, fix it immediately because someone else in your household may not see it.

Slippery steps and ladders would rank up on top of the list of causes of fall injuries. Aging carpets or decaying wood can grab a shoe or foot and send the victim sprawling in any direction. Falling from a height adds a new dimension of danger and potential injury. Forward falls can create facial or cranial injuries as well as whiplash to the neck and back. Landing hard on your tailbone on a hard step is very dangerous and can cause a fractured coccyx bone, compress a lumbar vertebra or herniated a lumbar disc. Always have good lighting and rails whenever possible. Fix or replace old carpet or flooring.

Review each room in your home independently. Visualize all activity that occurs in each room, how the furniture is arranged and make appropriate ergonomic changes to minimize future potential injuries.

Should an injury occur such as a back or joint trauma, as long as it is not life threatening, your Chiropractor would be a good first choice to help you.

Quote of the week: *"You must change in order to survive."*—Pearl Bailey

Proper positioning prevents back pain while driving

Question: My low back and neck are always sore after long car rides. How can I avoid back pain while driving distances?

Answer: There are many preventive measures you can take to avoid all types of back pain while driving distances:

Start with your own body. If you know you will be traveling a distance prior to your drive begin your day with stretching. I suggest Yoga as the primary way to prepare your mind, body, muscles and joints. Most importantly you should stretch your lower back, (gluteal) buttocks, and hamstring muscles because they will take on the extensive weight-bearing burden of driving.

Prepare for you trip ahead of time. Have proper directions and necessary information to avoid the stress of getting lost or confused. Bring healthy snacks such as nuts and dried fruit along with plenty of water.

Make your phone calls prior to your trip and avoid phone conversation while driving. I have seen a large increase in neck pain with patients that use car phones, especially those that are not hands free. Tilting your head to one side while talking and trying to look forward at the same time induces stress on neck muscles.

Posturally, make sure your car seat is comfortable and supports the lordotic (forward) curve of your low back. Your knees should be slightly higher than your waist. You elbow should from a 90-degree angle between your forearm and upper arm. Sitting too close or too far away from your steering wheel can stress your wrists.

Take breaks on long trips. Pull into rest stops or to the side of the road every two hours if necessary, to stretch, and walk for a while.

Your vehicle's seat should be supportive of your buttocks and low back. It should not sag to one side or be too soft that you sink down in it. The seat should be safe and functional so you can keep it upright and forward. The worst position while driving is leaning backward. All the weight bearing of sitting falls onto the lowest portion of your lumbar spine.

Be smart, be prepared, take breaks, and if your neck and back pain persist, see your local Chiropractor.

Quote of the week: *"You may not have been responsible for your heritage, but you are responsible for your future."*—Anonymous

Protect yourself from antibiotics

Question: I have been on antibiotics for various infections and every time I go on them I get stomach problems and feel I am worse off. What can I do to prevent the adverse effects of antibiotic usage?

Answer: Over utilization of antibiotics is at a national high. We are defeating ourselves by using antibiotics for most common colds and basic infections, many times when they are viral in origin.

The problem with antibiotics is that they don't have a special mission to kill just the invading bacterial organisms. Antibiotics kill all bacteria in their path, especially essential bacteria of the stomach lining as in your case. Over 150 million Americans will get a prescription for antibiotics this year. Besides breeding super bugs that will eventually make antibiotics inert, antibiotics kill the friendly bugs that live symbiotically within you.

Our bodies house some 400 species of friendly bacteria, or "probiotics". They cling to the walls of our stomachs and intestines. Friendly flora aid digestion, ward off pathogens and help us process folic acid and other critical nutrients. When the complex balance of microbes is jilted by stress, alcohol, antibiotics or poor nutrition, the consequences can be most unpleasant, ranging from stomachaches to vaginal infections, vitamin deficiencies, and chronic inflammation. Fortunately, a little fine tuning can keep your system humming.

We are not born with probiotics; they come from our environment. Babies encounter their first friendly microbes in breast milk. This is just one imperative reason we encourage our pregnant moms to nurse. Other sources of probiotics include yogurt, tofu (cultured milk) and miso (fermented soybeans). And because these microbes thrive on non-digested sugars called fructoligiosaccharides ("pro-biotics"), foods such as onions asparagus, tomatoes, garlic, artichokes, honey, and bananas can all help the bacteria thrive.

Scientists have long suspected a link between these microbes and overall health. Russian bacteriologist Ele Metchnokoff won a Noble Prize in the early 1990s for linking yogurt consumption to longevity. Drs. Sherwood Gorbach and Barry Goldoin of Tufts University discovered lactobacillus, the bacteria used in majority today's research.

Besides crowding out harmful bacteria, friendly flora maintain the acidic environment needed to control them, even releasing hydrogen peroxide to ward off wayward bugs. With less pathogens in our internal environment, the immune system is less likely to get overwhelmed. Studies show healthy bacteria word off bladder infections, vaginal infections, and even sexually transmitted diseases. Hospitalized infants, those given formula enriched with bifidoacteria (the bacteria found in breast milk) are less likely to develop infectious diarrhea.

Supplements of lactobacllus and probiotics are available through health food stores. Studies have shown that taking these supplements for two weeks prior to a typhoid vaccine exhibited a stronger immune response in those patients. More research proves that lactobacillus can lower the risk of respiratory infection in children.

Eat yogurt and probiotic foods and or take your probiotic supplements. Should you find yourself in need of more antibiotics in the future, do not take them at the same meal or they will negate each other.

Quote of the week: *"A man without a purpose is like a ship without a rudder."*—Thomas Carlyle

Psoas muscles keep our lower spine straight

Question: When my low back gets sore my entire pelvis leans over to one side. Why does this happen?

Answer: The leaning away from an irritation, especially in the spine, is called antalgic lean. When your body senses pain it tries to avoid it by shifting the pressure off the irritated area. We have patients walk in our office literally looking like question marks. The antalgic lean is a natural protective mechanism of the body to force us to avoid putting our weight onto the injured joint. The configuration of the vertebra of the spine is usually a wedge in the area of the antalgic lean. It is common to observe a disc bulge or disc herniation in magnetic-resonance imagings (MRIs) of the lumbar spine in these cases. These malpositions of the vertebra can also be seen on standard X-rays.

There are a set of muscles in your low back that play a significant role in the maintenance of your upright and symmetrical positioning of your lumbar spine. These muscles are called the psoas muscles and they originate along the upper lumbar and lower thoracic vertebra and attach deep in the body, to the anterior portion of your hip. There is one muscle coming off each side of your lower spine and they are like guide wires coming off at 45-degree angles. If one of these muscles is tighter than the other it will tug on the spine, pulling your entire body with it. These muscles work with other muscles in trying to adapt the spine to its irritation. If your low back demonstrates this type of deformity at any time, chances are you have a serious irritation and it should be immediately checked by a Chiropractor. A Chiropractor can examine the spine and determine the degree of irritation, as well as correct it in most cases. Balancing the psoas muscles and educating the patient on how to stretch these muscles is an essential means of correcting these antalgic lean conditions.

Quote of the week: *"Be kind, for everyone you meet is fighting a hard battle."*—Plato

Quality-of-life progress best assessed by patient

Question: What are the standards for measuring a patient's quality of overall health improvement after treatment at a doctor's office?

Answer: Standards for measuring quality of health improvement after a physician's treatment are based on a variety of factors. An initial assessment is essential to create a baseline of where the patient's health was at prior to care. To initiate a baseline, the present standards of care based on international studies from the World Health Organization (WHO), require the physicians office retrieve information subjectively from the patient.

The personal assessment of the patient's health by the patient is integral to create a common denominator when comparing mid-points and termination of treatment. Treatment should be based on both subjective assessments by the patient and objective findings by the doctor.

There are a number of different quality of life-assessment questionnaires available to utilize with patients. We use the Oswestry Health Assessment and S.F.36 forms in our offices. The S.F.36 has 36 questions and the Oswestry 25 questions. The questions asked in each are based on evaluating the patient's quality of life. Questions may include for example: How often does your pain occur? How is your condition interfering with interaction with your children? Is your sleep altered?

The bottom-line results of the information is to answer this question, "Is the intervention truly benefiting the overall health of the patient or are we just treating symptoms or having a minimum effect on this patient's life?"

Mid-way through care the patient will fill out the form to evaluate progress. If the scores of assessment indicate improvement, progress is being made and the protocol of care should be continued until maximal health in the eyes of the patient and doctor are achieved.

Quality of life studies look at the big picture and they are particularly valuable for Chiropractic care since it is designed to affect the entire person's ability to relate to their environment rather than the diagnosis and treatment of symptoms and disease.

Quote of the week: *"If we could make every moment in our lives count, that indeed would make for a long life."*—Anonymous

Reason for X-rays

Question: I was recently to a Chiropractor and part of my examination was X-rays. Does everyone that goes to a Chiropractor need X-rays and are they dangerous?

Answer: Technology has minimized the potential harm of radiation exposure during X-rays, significantly. Collimation is a tool utilized to only expose the necessary body part required for diagnostic study. Lead shielding reduces exposure to radiation sensitive areas. High-speed film and screens also reduce the time of exposure.

During a Chiropractic examination it is at the discretion of the Chiropractor to require X-rays or not. The basic premises behind X-rays are to view the patient's point of pain, determine potentially damaged bone like tissue or joints, and to avoid any risk to the patient from receiving treatment.

The Chiropractor uses the X-ray results in combination with many other diagnostic tests to come to a diagnosis as to where the origin of the patient's problem is. X-ray by itself is not an exact measure in determining a patient's condition.

There is risk and benefit in taking X-rays. If the doctor is going to make adjustments, he needs to know if there are any internal complications. If you are concerned about the exposure to radiation, you must weigh the risk against the benefits and make a decision. You have the right to deny X-rays but your doctor has the right to not treat you without them if he deems them necessary.

Your Chiropractor is aware of the hazards of X-rays. It is usually a year before follow-up X-rays are required. In acute distortion conditions such as severe whiplash, it may be necessary to re-X-ray within 6 to 8 weeks.

It is protocol to X-ray children with potential scoliosis to gauge the degree of distorted curvature change and monitor the child's growth. Pregnant women should never get X-rayed due to the potential exposure to the developing fetus. Always tell your doctor if you are pregnant or there's a chance you may be pregnant.

Quote of the week: *"None of us suddenly becomes something overnight, the preparations have been in the making for a lifetime."*—Gail Goodwin

Rib pains take time to heal

Question: I was in a car accident more than 18 months ago and my ribs still hurt, especially when I lift or even rub against anything. Is it normal for this to happen for so long?

Answer: Rib pain is considered the most intense and irritating pain a person can experience secondary only to facial pain.

The ribs form a protective shield for your internal organs including your heart, lungs, liver, pancreas and spleen. The ribs are attached by extremely strong criss-crossing fibers called intercostal muscles. Any insult (trauma) provoking these muscles causes an innate response for them to contract. Once contracted, the muscles pull together or approximate each rib so they create a solid bone mass as to protect the vital organs underneath them. The pain occurs because also lining each rib and running its entire length from anterior to posterior is the intercostal nerve.

These nerves, running bilaterally between every rib, are very sensitive to light touch and pressure. In the event of irritation they immediately send signals to the intercostal muscles to contract and elicit an excruciating pain response. This reaction is a means of telling you and your brain to stop what is creating a potential damage to your vital organs.

The reason the pain maintains a chronic nature is to continue the protective mechanism of preventing further injury.

Acute rib injuries require ice, rest and compression. X-rays are very important in severe injuries to differentially diagnose fractures. Magnetic-resonance imaging or computerized-tomography scan can help determine if there is internal organ damage.

Chronic problems such as yours can heal with appropriate nutritional supplementation, moist heat treatments and stretching. You may also require wearing a rib belt when doing aggressive activities to avoid re-exacerbation

Quote of the week: *"The greatest thing in this world is not so much where we are, but in what direction we are moving."*—O.W. Holmes

Roller-coaster rides

Question: My son wants me to go on the rides with him at the theme park. I am concerned about my spine. I have had car accidents and injuries to my neck elbow and back. Is it safe to go on roller-coaster type rides with a history of neck or back problems?

Answer: Many theme park rides are very traumatic to the body. We treat many patients that have had neck whiplash and low-back sprain and strain injuries on rides. This does not mean they are not safe. Most thrill rides require safety guidelines to prevent or minimize potential injuries to riders. Most rides have disclaimers on signs prior to riding, informing the public that they can create sudden and rapid movements to the body. Almost all rides inform potential riders that they should not get on if they are pregnant, suffer from heart conditions or have pre-existing medical conditions. Your pre-existing condition of neck or low-back pain should be examined by a competent physician such as a Chiropractor to determine potential additional injury or exacerbation.

Spending time with your child, doing something he or she enjoys, sometimes supercedes the fear of re-injuring your condition. Use common sense and if the ride looks like it is traumatic to the people on it, then avoid it. The most important idea is to have safe fun and quality time.

Quote of the week: *"Be grateful for luck but don't depend on it."*—Anonymous

Sciatica—Chiropractic best treatment

Question: What exactly is sciatica, and what is the best treatment for it?
Answer: Sciatica is the inflammation of the sciatic nerve, the largest and longest nerve in the body. Burning, sharp, piercing pain is the most common symptom felt in the low back extending to any part of the leg calf or foot. The sciatic nerve branches out and controls the organs in the pelvis including the reproductive system, bladder, kidneys and prostate. Abnormal symptoms caused by irritation from this large nerve may originally be in one of these organs or tissues, arise in the low back, legs or even the toes. You don't have to have pain running down your leg to have sciatica. Once irritated, coughing, sneezing sitting, standing or any basic movement can re-initiate symptoms.

Sciatica can frequently be caused by the misalignment of the joints of the spinal bones in the low back or pelvis, called vertebral subluxations. These misaligned spinal bones create pressure, choking on the nerves. This obviously interferes with the sciatic nerve's function. If the joint misalignment is left uncorrected, degeneration can begin to occur.

In the past, long periods of bed rest were commonly prescribed for sciatic pain and malfunction. Recent studies have confirmed that lengthy bed rest is a waste of time and may interfere with healing.

Another common prescription, epidural injections, does not help patients suffering from sciatica, either. Researchers in Germany did a 6-month study published this year in *Clinical Orthopaedics and Related Research*. These researchers found that spinal cortico-steroid injections do not help patients with sciatica improve any faster than those not given such injections.

What does seem to be the correct prescription is conservative Chiropractic adjustments to realign the misaligned vertebrae. According to the recently released United States Agency for Health Care Policy and Research (AHCPR) guidelines, "relief or discomfort can be accomplished most safely with Chiropractic adjustments."

Sciatica is a horrible experience and it doesn't just go away, even if the symptoms are dormant. Chiropractic care (sometimes coupled with simple exercises) normalizes the joint mobility, corrects the vertebral subluxation and takes pressure off the sciatic nerve. Correction of your sciatica could be as close as a call to your nearest Chiropractor.

Quote of the week: *"Courage is the price that life exacts for granting peace."*—Amelia Earhardt

Scooter injuries on the rise

Question: My son is constantly getting injured on his scooter. All the kids in the neighborhood ride them. I want him to be safe yet have fun. What can I do to protect him?

Answer: Scooter sales in the last year have more than doubled. Unfortunately, so has the number of emergency room visits for scooter-related injuries. According to a Reuter's report scooter-related injuries were nearly 18 times higher in September 2000 then in May 2000. Eighty five percent of reported accidents involve children below the age of 15; 23 percent of those were under the age of 8. The most common injuries are the arm and hand, 27 percent are to the head and face, and 24 percent are to the leg or foot. The spinal implications were not measured in these injury statistics. I personally see whiplash and sprain/strain injuries to the neck and or low back in most of the scooter injuries we have treated in our practice.

The Centers for Disease Control and Prevention and the Consumer Product Safety Commission recommend that all scooter riders wear helmets, knee, and elbow pads, and ride only in daylight on smooth, paved surfaces that have no traffic. Also, young children should be closely watched by an adult.

In the case of severe injuries, go to the emergency room, immediately. All children should be checked by a Chiropractor secondary to any scooter injury. The earlier restoration to normal balance of spinal structures occurs, the less likely pain and permanent injuries will remain.

Quote of the week: *"He who has health, has hope; and he who has hope, has everything."*—Proverbs

Seat-belt whiplash

Question: My girlfriend and I were in an auto accident and I was told I have seat-belt whiplash. What is seat-belt whiplash?

Answer: Seat-belt whiplash is a term used to describe an injury sustained secondary to the seatbelt tightening across your chest, shoulder, or neck due to an impact in your vehicle or possible an amusement park ride.

The term seat-belt whiplash describes the source of the problem (seat belt) and the result (whiplash). Whiplash is the rapid forward to back, back to forward or side to side motion of the upper torso or neck. The seat belt is designed to keep your upper body stationary, preventing you head from hitting a window or the dashboard. It does sacrifice you head, neck and shoulders which may whip forward at first, engaging the tightening action of the seat belt, then forcing these same regions to jolt back to where they originated (similar to the action of a whip).

The most common injury in the seat-belt whiplash is the shoulder and pectoral muscles, which lie directly under the position of the strap as it crosses your chest. Women, especially may experience bruising and laceration in severe impact accidents.

The whip like action of the belt can damage soft tissue directly under it or pull severely on your ligamentous and tendonous insertions into the ribs and shoulder joints. A torn rotator cuff is also a common injury in severe accidents.

The cervical spine which holds up your head, is the most prone to injury in a whiplash. The acceleration-deceleration action can cause a loss of the cervical lordosis (curve) in your neck leaving you with a barrage of symptoms ranging from headaches, neck pain, jaw pain, arm, wrist, and hand pain.

Any auto accident is a severe accident in my opinion. The mildest fender bender can create fractures, herniations and lifelong conditions.

The sooner your condition is examined and treated the less likely your may develop permanent injuries. Scar tissue builds up within 48 hours of an injury and the longer it persists without movement, the less likely it will totally heal.

I suggest both you and your girlfriend receive a Chiropractic evaluation to determine the severity of your condition. Chiropractors are experts in evaluating your spine for vertebral subluxations which are extremely common in auto accidents. Vertebral subluxations create neurological dysfunction which can create any or all the symptoms previously discussed.

Quote of the Week: *"In seeking happiness for others, you find it for yourself."*—Unknown

Seek care immediately with back pain

Question: I work at a factory and avoid reporting my back pain when it occurs on the job because of all the hassle I have to go through to get approval for treatment. What can I do to get treatment without going through the hassle?

Answer: An injury on the job should always be reported immediately to the proper authority in documenting the incident. Any witnesses should be included in the report for further verification. Not all injuries require lost time from neither work nor lost wages for temporary disability. My experience in working with Workers' Compensation and on the job injuries is that most employees want to be back at work as soon as possible and are not at all looking for a free paycheck. Unfortunately, employment in many cases is very skeptical of their employees taking advantage of an opportunity to miss work and get paid. This is a case of a few irresponsible people making it difficult for the majority of conscientious workers. This situation has created a hesitation on the employee to report minor injuries, especially back irritation because it is so common. The employer is also hesitant to respond quickly and efficiently in awarding time off and care because it is common. My advice is to always report any injury to your back while on the job as well as any back pain that occurs after you have left your job. Many injuries do not irritate you until hours or days after they have occurred. Reporting these conditions immediately after you experience pain is just as important as reporting them when they happen. Should permanent or partial permanent disability occur due to your back condition a detailed history will help in determining compensation and coverage for your treatment. Do not let anyone persuade you to not report an accident because it is minor or a hassle. The sooner you report your condition and have it treated the earlier you will get relief and prevent problems in the future.

A Chiropractor is an excellent solution to consider for your initial investigation to correct your back condition. Maintaining your spine prior to injury is better than waiting to get hurt at work. Consider an examination now, at your own convenience to determine the health of your back.

Quote of the week: *"A wise man learns from his experiences, but a wiser man learns from others' experiences."*—Peter Christakos

Self-help tips to help harness chronic headaches

Question: I go to a Chiropractor who helps me with my headaches. My question is, what can I do to help myself to prevent them?

Answer: Today, 90-percent of adults are affected by headaches. Causes can cover a broad range of reasons including diet, muscular tension, allergies, poor posture or stress—or headaches can be symptoms of underlying disease. Medical journals and medical books list literally hundreds of types of headaches and causes of them.

There are many specific actions you can take to prevent headaches. Here are a few:

- Avoid caffeine (chocolate, coffee, soda).

- Avoid food with high salt or sugar content.

- Seek to identify and eliminate any food allergies (a common cause).

- Get regular exercise—most importantly if you have a sedentary job. Exercise enough to sweat toxins and poisons out that build up in your system.

- Drink six to eight glasses of purified water daily.

- Get outside in the fresh air and sunshine at least one half-hour daily.

- Reduce or eliminate drugs or medications that you take regularly on your own.

- Try feverfew, ginko biloba, cayenne, or ginger for migraines. Supplement with B-complex vitamins, calcium and magnesium, and essential fatty acids (EFAs) daily.

- Learn a personal biofeedback technique such as meditation or yoga to give your mind rest from stress.

The most obvious solution I can give you, since headaches are one of the main reasons people seek Chiropractic care, is to continue your Chiropractic adjustments. Chiropractic care and advice will help. Relieving muscular tension and alleviating stress can be achieved by specific gentle spinal adjustments. A Chiropractor can advise you about posture, exercise, supplements, and relaxation techniques that will put you on the road to wellness.

Quote of the week: *"Somewhere, over the rainbow, skies are blue. And dreams that you dare to dream really do come true."*—from The Wizard of Oz

Sick and tired of being sick and tired?

Question: I always seem tired, foggy in the head and just run down. Rest and/or exercise do not help. What could be the problem?

Answer: Eliminating the potential cause of your condition as being organic such as a thyroid, adrenal or sugar problem, the most common cause of general malaise is an imbalanced nervous system. Your body is similar to a watch when it comes to maintaining a systematic fine-tuning to controlling our day's events. The watch and the body are both made up of hundreds of tiny parts, all of which must be meshed together in perfect coordination and balance, and with nothing to impede the flow of vital energy. The mainspring of the watch is the "brain." The human beings brain is the mainspring of all our actions, conscious and unconscious. Our system of interlocking gears, to transmit vital impulses from the brain, is our spinal cord.

Shock, fatigue, a fall or any of a hundred causes can throw the spine off balance, interfere with proper channeling of nerve impulses from the brain to the other organs of the body. When we are "run down," it's a symptom that, like our watches we need "adjusting." The Doctor of Chiropractic corrects the distortion that has altered or obstructed the proper channeling of nerve impulses, restoring the body to the desired equilibrium.

Quote of the week: *"The purpose of life is a life purpose."*—Robert Byrne

Side effects from adjustments are rare

Question: Is it possible to get side effects from Chiropractic adjustments?
Answer: Side effects are associated more with responses to taking medications than with Chiropractic adjustments. Most treatments are gentle and specific to the area of the spine associated with the dysfunction. The majority of patients treated by Chiropractors feel enhancement of their well being immediately following their adjustment.

Side effects or a reaction to treatment predominantly occurs in patients that are in acute pain. Acute pain patients present themselves in a state that requires a challenge to the Chiropractor to help them but not irritate the condition at the same time. Many of these type patients have severe muscle spasms and the only approach that will help them is to adjust into the area of the spasm and attempt to reduce the spasm first. It hurts initially no matter what the treatment. I don't condone the theory no-pain no-gain, however if the pain response is not interrupted the nervous system will continue its patterns of response to the patient's injuries.

A typical Chiropractic patient is going to be receiving treatment for more chronic distortions in their overall life functions or being treated for maintenance of their overall health and well being. Surveys of Chiropractic patients have indicated that a small portion of patients may experience headaches, stiffness, local discomfort, radiating discomfort, or fatigue secondary to a treatment. Re-localization of pain can indicate a rebalancing of weight bearing and the redistribution of nerve and/or blood supply to tissues that were improperly functioning. This implies that even in the small percentage of Chiropractic patients that have side effects to receiving these alterations in symptoms may be positive signs. These same patients that have side effects usually had them for a temporary period of 24 hours or less.

The bottom line is that Chiropractic is safe, effective and the most successful natural healing art in the world.

Quote of the week: *"Your integrity will affect your destiny: don't leave home without it."*—Anonymous

Simple healthy dieting guidelines

Question: There are so many diets, authorities and books telling us different ways to eat. I am confused about what is the best way to eat to stay healthy. What is your opinion on the basic guidelines to a healthy diet?
Answer: There are definite methods and protocols to eating healthy.

I will give you my guidelines to maintaining a healthy diet.

1. Eat a balanced meal within an hour after waking. This jump-starts your blood sugar and hormones.

2. Eat small, frequent meals. You will keep the fat burning process going, never feel hungry and prevent the high and low peaks of energy. Three balanced meals and two snacks a day with no more then 5 hours between meals is recommended.

3. Drink more water. Six to eight 10-ounce glasses per day is average for a 150-pound person.

4. Eat more fiber. Increase fruits and vegetable. Minimize pasta, cereals, breads, rice and potatoes.

5. Eat less fat in the form of fried greasy foods. Supplement with omega three fatty acids (including flax seed oil or fish oils).

6. Don't worry so much. If you blow your diet, you can start again at your next meal. The idea is to live better, not beat yourself up for making mistakes. We all learn this process the hard way.

7. Don't drink your calories. You can gain excess weight from high caloric drinks and ruin all your good work with your solid diet.

8. Stay adjusted. Chiropractors help maintain a healthy functioning nervous system which directly influences the balance of your digestive system.

To gain more information, read *The Zone* by Dr. Barry Sears. His book, *A Week in the Zone*, is a good book to start with. Another helpful book is *Eat Right for your Body Type* by Dr. Peter S. D'Adamo.

Quote of the week: *"Courage is the capacity to confront what can be imagined."*—Leo Roster

Sleep position for back health

Question: What is the best position for sleeping to keep your back healthy?

Answer: This is a common question I get in my office on a weekly basis. My patented answer is, any sleep that is deep and uninterrupted that leaves you feeling rested and rejuvenated is a great sleep session, regardless of the position you fell asleep or wake up in.

Hypothetically the best position to sleep is flat on your back with your hands at your side similar to a corpse. The neck should be supported either by a very thin pillow, no pillow or one that induces the cervical (neck) curve gently. This corpse position is considered the most favorable due to the natural anatomically posture of the entire body. Weight bearing for gravity is equally distributed from the head to the feet and the organs are at rest in their natural positions.

The second best position for sleeping would be the fetal position. This position as the name describes is lying on either side with both knees bent up towards the chest. The arms should once again be comfortable in front of the body. Placing a hand, arm or elbow under your head could potentially irritate neck, jaw, or shoulder muscles.

Utilization of large fluffy or over stuffed pillows is definitely a poor posture to place your head, neck and shoulders. Also, using two or three pillows in these same areas will aggravate the spine and neck region.

The worst position is lying on your stomach with you hands over you head, ironically the most common position my patients relate to me that they use. The reasoning behind this position being so unhealthy is that while on your stomach, your rib cage and torso are compressing your vital internal organs such as your heart, liver, lungs, spleen, etc. While compression is occurring to these organs they have less ability to contract and expand through normal phases of respiration. Blood supply and therefore oxygen supply may be inhibited or minimized not allowing normal daily detoxification and healing to occur fully.

Once again, despite any of the positions, it is most important to get a complete comfortable amount of sleep for normal healing and repair throughout the entire body.

If you suffer with insomnia and you sense it is not from emotional distress but from a physical ailment, then you should consult your Chiropractor regarding the nature or cause to your symptoms.

Quote of the week: *"Expect trouble as an inevitable part of life and repeat to yourself the most comforting words of all: This, too, shall pass."*—Ann Landers

Smoking increases low-back pain

Question: Can smoking cigarettes increase low-back pain?

Answer: For many years research could not identify all the adverse effects cigarette smoking has on our health. Research out of the journal *Medical Hypotheses,* 2001, evaluated the relationship between low-back pain and cigarette smoking. The results of the study indicate cigarette smokers have an increased risk of low-back pain, which may be caused by disc degeneration and spinal instability. There is evidence that disc degeneration of cigarette smokers is of more severe degree than non-smokers.

Cigarette smoking increases the release of specific proteolytic enzymes from the tiny capillaries in the lungs, which inhibits the protective proteins (protease). The high level of proteolytic (enzyme) activity of cigarette smokers speeds up the degenerative process. The study also implies that this activity also weakens the spinal ligaments resulting in spinal instability.

Cigarette smoking is absolutely dangerous to your health and can cause low-back pain.

Quote of the week: *"The secret of health for both mind and body is not to mourn the past, nor to worry about the future, but to live the present moment wisely and earnestly."*—Buddha

Spenoid bone stabilizes the skull

Question: My Chiropractor worked on a bone inside my mouth called the sphenoid bone. Why would he work on this and what does it do?

Answer: The sphenoid bone is a very important cranial bone found in your skull. It is flat and forms the roof of your hard palate inside your mouth. The sphenoid bone acts as an attachment site for many other bones and tissues. If you were to point all your fingers straight between your eyes at the bridge of your nose, that is approximately where your sphenoid bone sits. All the other cranial bones fit around this bone, making it very important to the symmetry and function of your entire skull and its contents, your brain. The most important supported structure by the sphenoid is the pituitary gland. Nicknamed the master gland, this pea-sized gland directly or indirectly controls the function of almost all the other glands in the body. The pituitary sits in a comfortable little pocket called the sella tursica, which is located right between your eyes at the bridge of your nose. When the sphenoid bone becomes displaced or irritated the sella tursica can move minutely, enough to affect the pituitary gland adversely, which in a cascading chain of events can cause a barrage of symptoms ranging from visual disturbance to energy fatigue. Besides, pituitary dysfunction, other conditions created by the displaced sphenoid include TMJ disorders, sinus conditions, and facial pain.

Your Chiropractor would want to correct the sphenoid after determining other priority treatments did not correct your problem. It is basically painless to correct a dropped sphenoid bone. It is done by pushing up on the roof of the mouth while the patient assists with correct phases of respiration. A corrected sphenoid bone can give immediate relief to many of the symptoms already mentioned.

Quote of the week: *"Dream and dare to be different!"*—K. Sarginson

Spinal stretching reduces back pain

Question: What exercise would you suggest for back pain that is everywhere in my spine? Does stretching really help reduce pain?

Answer: Daily spinal stretching is essential for reduction of pain in a sore back or maintenance of a healthy spine. Our modern day lifestyle trends predispose us to excessive sitting, especially at the computer. Our busy schedules and increased travel reduces the potential time we can prioritize to exercise. A healthy spine is a healthy attitude and happier more pain free life. Your entire disposition can be determined by how healthy you feel on any given day. You can choose to make a difference in your own physiology, which in turn will improve your emotional attitude and degree of fulfillment.

Incorporating a stretching regimen to your daily routine will be the greatest asset to a successful lifestyle you could ever make. If you never stretched or exercised before, starting with small increments of time and challenge is the most intelligent method of incorporating a stretching program. Simple knee to chest stretches, individually and then together for ten seconds, each time for three repetitions is the easiest and first basic stretch to start. This is done while lying on your back in bed or on the floor. Additional progressive stretches can be incorporated as the comfort levels are reached. Always challenge yourself but never push yourself into pain. There is a fine line between pain and a good stretch.

Always consult your Chiropractor first before starting your spinal stretching program. Continuous or severe pain is a contra-indication to performing any particular stretch. Yes, you can injure yourself by doing a stretch that is too extreme for your particular condition. Have goals and vision while doing your routine. Learn about what each muscle is responsible for in your movements.

Procrastination is the number one way of not initiating a stretching program. It is easy! Ultimately, investing 20 minutes of your morning doing spinal stretching will give the remainder of your entire day a new happier complexion.

Quote of the week: *"To wish to progress is the largest part of progress."*—Lucious Annaeus Seneca

Spine develops first and controls all functions

Question: Why do Chiropractors place so much emphasis on the spine and nervous system?

Answer: The answer to this question is the premise behind the entire foundation and philosophy of Chiropractic. To understand why the spine and the central nervous system (CNS) are so vital we must first have a quick lesson in human embryology.

Fertilization occurs when a male sperm penetrates an active ovum (egg) leading to mitosis (multiplication of cells). The multiplying cells amass themselves to become a morula (clusters of cells). At this point differentiation and specialization occurs. This means each cluster of cells starts to get its own identification. Some become liver cells, some become heart cells, some become kidney cells, etc. At approximately six weeks something remarkable occurs. All the cells line up and down the fetus creating something called a primitive streak. This primitive streak becomes your spine and CNS. The spine is the first, primary and most important organ in your body, from six weeks of our inception and throughout the remainder of our lives.

From this moment on the spine will dictate how we grow and heal. Your spine and brain—the CNS, design all information to every organ, tissue, and cell in your body. It would make a lot of sense to keep the CNS in as close to perfect order as possible for your entire life. Because the spine is so vital, Chiropractors dedicate their careers to helping patients maintain the maximum potential of their spines, knowing that if the spine is healthy, all other functions of the body can be maximized. This is the reason Chiropractors treat pregnant women and infants. The earlier spinal dysfunction is discovered the less likely dysfunction will occur in growth and development. Chiropractors believe in preventive exams throughout a child's life and into adulthood, prior to symptoms occurring.

The amazing part about your spine and its development is that all this occurs without any help from anything but nature. The innate intelligence given to mankind creates the body and heals the body. Chiropractors help maintain the balance so everything goes right. The body was made to be perfect, above, down, and inside-out.

Quote of the week: *"The secret of life is enjoying the passage of time."*—James Taylor

State Workers' Compensation laws need changes

Question: I injured my low back at work and wanted to see a Chiropractor but was refused by the Workers' Compensation doctors. Why doesn't Workers' Compensation recognize Chiropractic for work-related injuries?
Answer: Welcome to the great state of New Jersey. Our state, along with a handful of other states, remains archaic and prejudiced in relationship to employees' rights to choose their own physicians in cases of work-related injuries. As the law is written, the Workers' Compensation insurance carrier has the right to direct treatment, diagnostic testing and services to the physicians and facilities of their choice. Unfortunately, my clinical experience and interactions with these companies indicate that the majority of these physicians and facilities have a greater interest in cost containment for the insurance company they work for rather than the health and welfare of the injured employee. Since these facilities and physicians work for the insurance company there is a built-in vested interest to maintain job security. Most every other state in the country reversed these laws to protect the injured employee and employer. Your employer doesn't even have a say in the matter once it goes to the Workers' Compensation insurance carrier.

The ironic situation with the Workers' Compensation physicians not referring to Chiropractors is that all studies indicate that treatment costs, lost work days and compensation paid workers with musculoskeletal injuries is substantially less for those injured workers going to Chiropractors versus medical doctors. Patient satisfaction was much higher also. A study done in North Carolina extensively studied 96,927 claims between 1975 and 1994 and was published in the September 2004 edition of the *Journal of Manipulative and Physiological Therapeutics.*

My suggestion is to write your state representatives and demand support to change this dictatorship in the Workers' Compensation insurance industry.

Quote of the week: *"When nothing is sure, everything is possible."*—Margaret Drabble

Straight look at curve balls

Question: My son is 11-years-old and pitches for his baseball team. I am concerned he may injure his shoulder because he is throwing curve balls. Is it advisable to have a child this young throw curve balls?

Answer: As a coach, father, and Chiropractor with 12-and 14-year old sons that are baseball players, I will advise you in each category.

As a coach you want a child to learn the fundamentals of pitching first. A proper pitching motion puts minimal stress on the body and simultaneously allows for efficient reproducible accuracy and speed change. Many professional pitchers choose not to throw curve balls because of the mechanics and its effect on their shoulders, arms, and wrists.

As a father my priorities are my children's safety, learning and having fun. If mastering a curve at this age is in any way interference with proper learning and enjoyment, it is not worth pushing the issue.

As a Chiropractor with 24-years experience of treating sports injuries to young athletes, I would always say absolutely no to curve balls even into the high school years. This can be considered a controversial position but my opinion is based on clinical experience.

My reasoning is based on the fact that at as late as even 17 years old, the secondary growth plates are not totally solidified. There is potential continued growth. The tendons and ligaments of the shoulder, elbow and wrist attach to the boney extensions around the growth plates. Excessive torque as in the rotating action of the wrist and elbow in a curve ball pitch can over stress these insertions of the ligaments and tendons near the growth plates. A damaged growth plate can cause a permanent disfigurement to the joint as well as functionally damaging the joint.

The shoulder is surrounded by a rotator cuff of four muscles inserting into the same boney protrusion. A disruption of this joint can irritate any of these four muscles.

The best protocol of a dad, or coach helping his son or daughter learn to pitch, is use safety and fundamentals first. Never force a child to continue a motion if they complain of pain or discomfort. Ask yourself if the motion looks fluent and comfortable. Ask your child if the motion feels fluent and comfortable. Don't add additional pitches until your child masters the basic pitches.

If you child is injured or in pain consider a Chiropractor as a primary treating physician for their sports injury.

Quote of the week: *"There is no security in life, only opportunity."*—Mark Twain

Summer sports require warm ups

Question: Every summer I start playing volleyball and tennis and every summer I injure something else. Am I doing something wrong or am I just injury prone?

Answer: The warm weather prompts many of us in the north to return to the field or court. Whether it is to get in shape, be more competitive, or just have fun and enjoy the great outdoor sunshine, it is all good. Two thirds of all sports injuries are a result of attempting too much too fast. Below are five of the most common sports injuries and how to prevent them:

1. Knee injury: Workout on the softest surface possible. Wear proper footwear, with soft flexible soles, and when jumping, land with your knees bent.

2. Muscle soreness: Allow for a warm-up and cool-down period. Do the appropriate stretches for the muscles you will you use in that activity. Don't overdo it! Pushing yourself when you feel spent is a common time for tearing muscle tissue.

3. Side stitch (sharp pain or cramp under the rib cage): Practice proper breathing. Don't "work through" pain. Stop and walk slowly. Don't eat and immediately perform vigorous exercise.

4. Shin splints (mild to severe ache in front of lower leg): Progressively strengthen muscles in this region. Keep your calves well stretched.

5. Blisters: Wear shoes and socks that fit well. Wear preventive taping, if necessary. Avoid wearing moist or wet footwear or socks.

Any injury that remains persistent should be checked by your Chiropractor. Non-invasive, natural care that deals with the cause of your condition is a prudent first choice for your healthcare.

Quote of the week: *"Today's preparation determines tomorrow's achievement."*—Anonymous

Tai Chi is the perfect exercise for elderly

Question: I am in my early 80s and would like to exercise but my joints are weak and painful. What exercise or activity would you suggest for someone my age?

Answer: The best exercise for the elderly that avoids additional strain and injury is Tai Chi. Millions of people in China, especially the elderly, practice Tai Chi on a daily basis. Tai Chi is a slow motion martial art that builds and strengthens agility and balance. It looks like a cross between shadow boxing and slow motion ballet.

Tai Chi combines intense mental focus with deliberate, graceful movements that allow balance to improve which is especially important to the elderly. Anyone practicing Tai Chi regularly expresses the spiritual and psychological benefits.

Like yourself, many older men and women are healthy but relatively inactive. This art fills the void. It takes a few months to reap the effects of Tai Chi, but when you do your lifestyle, mental, and physical balance will be greatly enhanced.

There are many good how to books to get you started, or you can choose from among the growing number of classes offered at recreation centers and health clubs in our area. Performing Tai Chi with a group or a trainer will help develop proper performance as well as increase potential to stick with it.

Should your health allow more agility, combining a walking program to maintain cardiovascular conditioning would compliment the Tai Chi.

I admire and respect your desire to maintain your health. Your wisdom regarding the prevention of illness through exercise is a dynamic model for others your age to follow.

Quote of the week: *"There is a time to let things happen, and a time to make things happen."*—Hugh Pratner

Teeth grinding at night is a sign of imbalance

Question: My husband grinds his teeth at night and it is annoying. His teeth are even wearing down. He doesn't think it is a problem but I am concerned. Why does he do this and can you help?

Answer: The most common cause of grinding your teeth is a temporal-mandibular joint imbalance (TMJ), also commonly known as the jaw. The name comes from the muscles above the jaw the temporalis. This fan shaped muscle is thin as paper and runs along the side of your skull.

When you bear down on your teeth and hold a finger to your skull just above your ear you can feel it contract. Along with the masseter muscle below your jaw joint, these two muscles make up your muscles of mastication and together are the strongest muscles in the body based on size per tensile contraction. Grinding the teeth at night is a secondary result of minor contractions of these two muscles.

Anxiety can prevent the relaxation of these muscles causing tension even while sleeping. Another cause is sinus congestion. Engorged sinus cavities in the face stimulate the jaw muscles to contract to squeeze out the over accumulated fluid, once again causing the teeth to shift back and forth. The most common cause of teeth grinding also medical defined as bruxing, is an imbalance structurally of the TMJ. Dental conditions may force a high side to develop. As a person opens their mouth it deviates to one side or the other. The jaw may even make an "S" motion as it opens. Another sign of imbalance is the inability to open wide enough to get three knuckles inside. Many dentists are capable of working with dental and height imbalances of the TMJ. Should the condition persist, Chiropractic is a very viable solution. Balancing cranial sutures with muscle balancing techniques is effective along with spinal adjustments of the upper cervical spine and occiput.

The TMJ is a very sensitive joint, due to its proximity to the brain. Because of the high concentration of neurons it is extremely painful when injured and can cause symptoms all over the entire body.

Teeth grinding is a serious sign of imbalance and should be attended to with or without immediate symptoms.

Quote of the week: *"Learn as if you would live forever, live as if you would die tomorrow."*—Mahatma Ghandhi

Tennis elbow solution

Question: I am an avid tennis player but have been hampered by severe tennis elbow as of recent. I have tried ointments and every tennis elbow support on the market, still without relief. Is there anything a Chiropractor can do?

Answer: Yes, Chiropractic is very beneficial for most tennis elbow conditions. Tennis elbow, also known as elbow tendinities or epicondylits, means there is an inflammation in the area where a tendon attaches one of the forearm muscle to the bone of the upper arm.

Symptoms include inflammation, elbow pain, and wrist weakness. You don't have to play tennis to get tennis elbow. Many cumulative traumas are the result of repetitive motions in sports such as tennis and golf. These game repetitive motions may be performed in workplace, office or factory. Tennis elbow can recur because there is not sufficient nerve supply necessary to rebuild healthy elbow tissue. Misalignment of the relationship of the two forearm and upper arm bones can also create the same inflammatory process.

Chiropractors work to restore normal blood supply that helps the healing process and will educate you in proper stretching and strengthening techniques. Some patients require supportive devices to minimize discomfort during or when away from their activity which re-creates the condition.

Quote of the Week: *"Believe only half of what you see and nothing that you hear."*—Dinah Mulock Craik

Tingling/numb extremities have multiple causes

Question: I get tingling and numbness in the extremities. I have been to many different doctors and everyone gives me a different diagnosis. Why is this a difficult condition to figure out?

Answer: Tingling and numbness are symptoms that many conditions create. Isolating which of the many causes it could be is not as simple as it may appear. These symptoms can be musculoskeletal or organic in nature. This means it can come from a joint, muscle or ligament problem or an organ-related referred pain such as the heart. An average healthy person can wake up with tingling and numbness in his/her hands after sleeping with an arm under her/her head and disturbing circulation to an extremity. The opposing extreme would be a person suffering with diabetic neuropathy that is resulting in permanent loss of blood and neurological distribution to the extremities causing death to tissues. The numbness and tingling can become permanent and loss of enervation lead to gangrene requiring the removal of the tissue that is necrosed. I have found that the range of causes lies somewhere between these two extremes.

As a Chiropractor we treat many conditions such as yours, which are directly related to the interruption of nerve supply to the extremity or extremities in question. A pinched nerve or vertebral subluxation at the level of the spine can interrupt nerve flow to its endpoints. When a light bulb goes out in your home it would be prudent to first check the bulb itself, but if the bulb was not broken the next best place would be to check the source of power to that bulb, such as the fuse box. The spine is the fuse box of the body and when there are problems with an extremity it is important to check that extremity and/or symptom. If there is not a problem in that extremity the next best place to check is the spinal level or fuse that returns the power to that extremity.

Chiropractors are similar to electricians in that we both turn the power back on. The difference is the body is a living self-healing organism and will repair itself once the power is returned. Any recurrent symptoms of tingling/numbness are serious signs that should be checked immediately by your physician whether a Chiropractor or M.D. Any history of heart disease or diabetes should be relayed to your doctor. If you have a prior history of trauma whether serious or repetitive, as in carpal tunnel syndrome, it should be investigated.

Quote of the week: *"Nature, time, and patience are the three greatest physicians."*—Proverb

Tips to stay young in your 40s

Question: I am in my early 40s and want to maintain a fit and healthy lifestyle as possible. What areas of my daily and weekly activities should I focus on?

Answer: The 40s are traditionally a time when people begin to re-evaluate their lives, and when many Americans begin to worry about aging. Staying young means embracing the positive aspects of aging. In many eastern cultures growing old with dignity and joy is a blessing. Accepting where we are in the passage of life can be the most enriching experience of all.

You may want to take preventative heath measures regarding any family histories of health problems. Tests to consider if your family history includes disease are colonoscopies, prostate screenings, mammograms, and any heart disease related exams.

Your muscle mass begins to decline in your 40s and even if your weight has relatively been unchanged in 20 years you should add muscle-building strength exercises to your fitness regimen.

Examine your attitude toward aging. Recognize that middle age has its benefits, such as having more time to focus on your own interests as your children become more independent or you just gain more free time in general. Nurture yourself by striving to reach your goals and by maintaining a relaxed attitude toward life.

Nutritionally, studies indicate that middle age is an appropriate time to add soy products like soybeans and tofu to your diet. Soy can help protect against prostate cancer and potential irritants that accompany menopause.

Maintain a healthy nervous system with periodic Chiropractic adjustments. Drink plenty of water and get adequate rest.

Quote of the week: *"Experience is not what happens to you; it is what you do with what happens to you."*—Aldous Huxley

Tubes for ear infections may be avoided

Question: Both of my children have had middle-ear infections and drainage tubes were used for my first child without any effect. My younger child has the same problem and I would like to know if there is anything besides tubes to help?

Answer: Earache is the most common reason after well-baby and child-care, for visits to a doctor. Unfortunately, current medical treatment for middle-ear problems has been less than adequate in most cases. There are multiple factors that contribute to the possible cause of middle-ear infections in newborns and children. Prior to using medications and tubes, there are alternative approaches.

Determining the cause of the middle-ear infection can be significant in determining the solution, especially in recurrent conditions. The cause can come from allergies, many times from cow's milk products, wheat (gluten), soy, corn, peanuts, and others. Another cause is infection from bacteria or viruses. If the cause is bacteria and it has been confirmed with a swab sample, antibiotics may be warranted. Be careful, for overuse of and inappropriate use of antibiotics may lead to problems such as antibiotic-resistant bacteria. Another possible cause of middle-ear infections is mechanical obstruction. Some doctors have suggested that changes in spinal, cranial, and jaw (TMJ) bio-mechanics may contribute to the development of middle ear problems in children. Alteration in bio-mechanics may occur due to trauma before or at birth, from a fall or accident, or from other influences. In addition, the Eustachian tube in children has not yet reached an angle for optimal drainage. Newborn's and children's Eustachian tubes run parallel to the ground or horizontal and as we develop the tube angles vertically downward for easier and more natural drainage.

Some feeding positions may encourage flow into the tubes, and mechanical disturbances can further impede drainage.

Spinal manipulation, cranial balancing, and TMJ therapy may be effective in treating some cases of acute and chronic middle-ear effusion (leaking fluid). Besides the above, dietary and nutritional changes to assist the immune system are important. Psychological stress and environmental factors also may play a role.

Complementary treatments and natural remedies are a great opportunity to help your children in many cases.

Quote of the week: *"It is not who is right, but what is right, that is important."*—Thomas Huxley

U.S.A. has a mental-health crisis

Question: I have been suffering with mental-health problems for years and felt very private about my condition with friends and family. I am just finding out now that a good portion of my friends and family are suffering with mental disorders also. A few of them tell me their Chiropractors help them with their conditions. Is this true?

Answer: Not everyone is going crazy but after I give you the following statistics you might believe it. According to the U.S. Surgeon General: About one in five Americans will suffer from a mental disorder in the course of a year. Approximately 18.8 million American adults suffer from depression. Treatment costs run about $80 billion a year.

Mental illness causes more disability and loss of life than any other illness except heart disease. Cost of the resulting loss in productivity is estimated at $80 billion per year. Cost-effective treatments now exist for many forms of mental illness.

Mental illness is an illness like other illnesses. Covering it up and avoiding dealing with the cause of the illness is unhealthy in itself. You are not alone when it comes to feeling embarrassed and private by your feelings. I believe that we all experience highs and lows in our emotional states and what makes each of us different is how we cope with these changes.

Uncontrollable circumstances exuding large magnitudes of stress can trigger long-term mental disease. Low-grade continuous mild stress can affect us in the same way. Many theories contest that mental illness is a chemical imbalance and or genetic trait. One correlation that I have observed is that when a mentally fragile person has additional stress, such as physical trauma, they are subject to an exacerbation of their mental illness. Reduction of their physical stress allows a mentally challenged person to deal more directly with their illness. Chiropractors definitely help their mentally ill patients in this way. Balancing the nervous system also balances brain activity since the two are inseparable.

Quote of the week: *"As you go the way of life you will see a great chasm. Jump. It is not as wide as you think."*—Native American Proverb

Visualization therapy

Question: I am a cancer survivor and utilized visual therapy to heal. Can using this therapy enhance spinal corrections?

Answer: I personally am a strong advocate of conceptual/visual therapy. Many Chiropractors and other healers simultaneously utilize the same principals like you as a patient.

Your brain can be programmed to respond to conditions. Installing programs that reverse detrimental illness are very real and successful methods of combating mental and physical illness.

Conceptual healing educates the patients to see themselves as healing or totally free of their disease state.

It is not the cure by any means and should never be substituted for appropriate medical or Chiropractic treatment. We can convince the body and mind to enhance it's responses to the healing process by visualizing each step of the healing process in a clear, precise, active state. The more specific and educated the patient is in their conceptualizing, the more effective they can create the re-patterning and improvement of their condition. An example is a cervical spine whiplash patient who would envision increased mobility in their cervical vertebrae, soft, flexible smooth, contracting neck muscles with a warm flow of gentle calmness to the surrounding soft tissue. The greater the amount of these senses utilized the more effective in assisting the brain and treatment.

Your Chiropractor can enhance the effect of their treatment to you by envisioning the same result, as they adjust your spine.

What you can conceive, you can achieve. How you see yourself and how you feel can be a mirror image. Take a chance, look at your reflection and start looking at yourself as healthy. It just might happen.

Quote of the week: *"There can be no happiness if the things we believe in are different from the things we do."*—Freya Madeline Stack

Vitamin supplement content can be deceiving

Question: I take a lot of vitamin supplements yet I don't feel I am getting the benefits from them. What makes one vitamin supplement better than another?

Answer: The FDA presently has loose restrictions on vitamin manufacturers' labels.

The loose restrictions are that contents are listed but absorption rates and the ability to breakdown the supplement after digested are not listed. The outer coating, nor how the supplement is (adhering) to form its shape are not always listed. Many less effective supplements are produced with glucose (sugar) coatings which give the shiny appearance to the exterior surface. In these supplements breakdown and absorption will unlikely not occur in the gut wall where most of the benefit occurs. Multi-vitamins classically are produced in this manner. Sugar or carbohydrate type coatings can also be very allergic to many people, not only preventing nutritional value but also irritating the stomach.

The closer to natural food the supplements is the greater its absorption and nutritional value. Avoid supplements with sugars, food colorings, and artificial ingredients and that may be allergenic.

Nutritionists, Chiropractors and homeopathic physicians have training in nutrition and can guide you to appropriate supplementation, if needed.

The best way to get great nutritional supplementation is to eat properly and you will not need vitamin supplements at all.

Quote of the week: *"The indispensable first step to getting the things you want of life is this, decide what you want."*—Ben Stein

Weekend warrior

Question: I am a weekend warrior with sports. I play softball on the weekends and want to know if stretching really makes a difference?

Answer: The answer is a resounding yes, especially for the weekend warrior.

You are typical of the average adult athlete. Whether it is two or seven days a week that you work out, stretching is imperative to prepare for activity, prevent injury and cool down muscles after working them.

It only takes approximately 15 minutes to appropriately stretch prior to physical activity. Stretching is essential because it elongates the muscles prior to use. An unprepared muscle that is given a rapid stretch will pull from its origin and insertion around the bone it attaches to.

The end points of muscles are tendons and their responsibility is to attach to bone.

When the muscles vigorously pulls at these tendons they move the bone to quickly causing a "strain" at this region.

A strain is accompanied by swelling, restriction of movement and pain.

Pre-stretching the muscle and tendons prepares the tissue for sudden, quick jolts by elongating the tendons' insertions.

Pre-stretching prior to a jolt is less likely to cause a strain because there is more length to the tendon to adapt to the movement. Stretching also prevents injuries to the belly of the muscle. The belly of the muscle contains fluid. A cooler fluid moves slower and adapts slower to movement. Stretching warms out the stagnate cooler fluids in the belly and dissipates toxins such as lactic acid that accumulate secondary to dormancy.

A well-prepared muscle means a well-prepared joint. The joints that are predominantly used for your particular activity should be concentrated on, although full-body stretching is always recommended.

A well-prepared body includes a well-prepared nervous system. Many athletes choose Chiropractic care to enhance their performance. The nervous system controls muscle function and if you continue to feel tight or sore in your muscular regions you should consult a Chiropractor to determine if assistance is required.

Quote of the Week: *"Failure is not the worst thing in the world... The very worst is not to try."*—Unknown

Whiplash can occur from injuries other than auto accidents

Question: I recently slipped and almost fell but didn't hit my head. My neck was very sore and when I went to the Chiropractor he said it was a whiplash injury. Is this possible?

Answer: Whiplash is most commonly associated with car accidents but it may also result from everyday accidents like yours. "Whiplash" itself is a term used to describe the condition caused when, as a reaction to unexpected force, your head springs backwards as your body moves forward, and then as it recoils, your head springs forward. Whiplash may also happen in reverse order with the head moving forward as the body moves backward, and from side impacts. Symptoms of whiplash include pain in the neck, shoulders, and arms; stiffness; headache; dizziness; visual disturbances; nausea; sore throat; trouble swallowing; loss of voice; insomnia; and others.

Some of the more common causes of whiplash include: car accidents, slips and falls, and sudden head movements. Your head may be more prone to whiplash because of the following: Lifting things incorrectly, hereditary weakness, gradual wear and tear, various medical conditions, poor posture, fatigue, and stress.

Considering that your head weighs approximately 10 pounds, balances on a stack of vertebrae, and moves about with the help of your neck and shoulder muscles, it is surprising that its is not injured more frequently. When it is injured, however, how do you differentiate the times when you need a Chiropractic treatment versus simple rest? You would be wise to seek treatment if you have symptoms of whiplash, or your pain lasts longer than 24 hours. Seek treatment immediately if you have pain that is worsened by sneezing, coughing or laughing. Also seek help for any pain accompanied by nausea, vomiting, dizziness, numbness, or other unusual and worrying symptoms.

Chiropractic care is structured with all the components necessary to diagnose and treat a mild or severe whiplash condition.

Quote of the week: *"It's what you learn after you know it all that counts."*—John Wooden

You can prevent your own back pain

Question: How can I prevent my own back pain?

Answer: Many patients and friends ask me how they can prevent back pain or how they can stop the back pain from coming back once it is healed. The best answer is common sense. We tend to perform activities or perform work well beyond our personal capacities. Know your limits regarding length of time you can sit, stand, lift, twist, etc. Know your endurance limits, so that once they are exhausted, you don't act insufficiently or make mistakes with your back.

Some other basic tips are: Don't lift by bending over. Instead, bend your hips and knees and then squat to pick up the object. Keep your back straight, and hold the object close to your body. Don't twist your body while lifting. The joints of your spine are designed for one movement at a time. Multiple combined repetitive movements can irritate the back. Push rather than pull, when you must move heavy objects. If you must sit for long periods, take frequent breaks and stretch. Put a phone book or stool under one foot to remind you not to sit forward while working at a computer or desktop. Wear flat shoes or shoes with low heels. Don't wear large wallets in your back pocket or heavy pocket books over your shoulders.

Exercise regularly a minimum of three times a week for 20 minutes. Stretch on a daily basis. An inactive lifestyle leads to weak muscles in the back.

Most importantly see your Chiropractor on a regular basis to determine if you need a preventative maintenance adjustment. The worst thing that could happen is you won't need a treatment that day and you know you spinal health is perfect.

Quote of the week: *"Everything counts! Everything you do helps or hurts, adds up or takes away."*—Brian Tracy

Youth back pain common, but not normal

Question: My son seems to always complain of mid-back pain even when he isn't playing sports. He is 14, healthy and fit. Is it normal for teenagers to get back pain?

Answer: Back pain is prevalent among school-aged youth. A study of students in Denmark surveyed 481 children aged 8 to 10 years, and 325 adolescents aged 14 to 16 years. The findings showed 39-percent had thoracic (mid-back) pain for at least one month. Thoracic pain is most common in childhood, whereas thoracic pain and lumbar pain (low-back) are equally common in adolescence. Neck pain and pain in more than one area of the spine are rare in both age groups. No gender differences were found.

Although these areas of the spine are the most common to each of these age groups. It is not normal for a child or adolescent to have any back pain. Developed back pain in a youth without any predisposing factors is a strong indicator to have your child's spine checked by a spinal expert such as a Chiropractor. Back pain after an injury obviously should be examined. The fact is that a periodic check of your child's spine is probably the best preventative measure you can take as a parent to protect your child's health.

Quote of the week: *"To the world you may be one person, but to one person you may be the world."*—Anonymous

978-0-595-37366-6
0-595-37366-6